SO YOU'RE
THINKING OF GOING TO
A CHIROPRACTOR

Other Keats Books
of Relevant Interest

So you're thinking of going to a chiropractor

ROBERT DRYBURGH, D.C.

Foreword by A. Earl Homewood, D.C.

KEATS PUBLISHING, INC. New Canaan, Connecticut

The information in this book is not intended as medical advice. Its intention is solely informational and educational. It is assumed that the reader will consult a medical or health professional should the need for one be warranted.

Library of Congress Cataloging in Publication Data

Dryburgh, Robert.
 So you're thinking of going to a chiropractor.
 1. Chiropractic—Popular works. I. Title.
RZ244.D78 1984   615.5'34   83-81049
ISBN 0-87983-345-9

Printed in the United States of America

Keats Publishing, Inc., 27 Pine Street (Box 876)
New Canaan, Connecticut 06840

Contents

Preface

This book has been prepared for the chiropractic patient who has not studied the body extensively, but who is faced with the question of how to prepare for a healthy future. In it is information that a chiropractor would like to share with his patients if he had time and opportunity.

Patients who have experienced the benefits of chiropractic care are often motivated to tell their chiropractic experience, but they do not understand how or why chiropractic helped them. The scope of chiropractic, beyond their particular problem, is still a mystery to them.

I would like to talk about chiropractic as we see it from the inside. If a little of the excitement of being part of a dynamic and growing profession sparkles here and there in the narrative, it is because being a chiropractor has not lost its fascination for me. I'm still amazed every day in the office that the results are so often much better than I would have predicted.

Let's take a look at present-day chiropractic science.

Robert Dryburgh, D.C.

This book is dedicated to my wife Joy, who has been my chiropractic assistant for years. She has listened to me as I presented these principles over and over to patients in the office and motivated me to write this book for the help and encouragement of others.

Foreword

An invitation to write a foreword to an interesting, layman-oriented, informative book relative to chiropractic is an honor and privilege which cannot be ignored or taken lightly by one now on the sidelines of the chiropractic profession.

Dr. Dryburgh has given the reader the opportunity to explore this relatively new subdivision of generic medicine, with emphasis on those areas of personal interest for the average layman, the maintenance and restoration of health. However, the professional will find much of interest and information that may not have been acquired elsewhere. Beginning with a brief discussion of fetal development to aid in visualizing the human as a unit of structure and function, and continuing with an introduction to the chiropractic physician as a person, the highlights of history of the profession and its aims and objectives, several of the areas of specialization and the research efforts, past, present and future, the text carries the reader along in an interesting manner, with many examples of patients and their problems to which many readers may be able to relate, and the results that may be expected in similar conditions. To present such a vista of a profession is challenging, but Dr. Dryburgh rose to the occasion in a masterly manner.

It must be understood that such an introduction to the second largest school of generic medical thought must mirror the particular interests and field of specialization of the writer; another practitioner undertaking a similar presentation would demonstrate quite a different emphasis. The founder of chiropractic, D. D. Palmer, pointed out clearly in his writings that subluxations are the result of mechanical, chemical, and/or psychological environmental stress, and chiropractors have differed widely in their individual areas of interest and expertise. Dr. Dryburgh emphasizes the mechanical stresses and injuries which create structural disrelations, dysfunctions and subluxations and their somatic symptoms. Another doctor might well have stressed the chemical causes, need for environmental correction and restoration of the structural integrity of the individual patient. Another would perhaps emphasize the psychological causes of muscular hypertension and subsequent disrelations with their neurological disturbances. One with a greater interest in the dysfunctions of the internal organs which require the diagnostic workup, X-rays of viscera, laboratory investigation, and so on, with the added interest in the structural disrelations which alter the neural supply, would discuss this subject from yet another point of view. Chiropractic is a very complex subject, and no practitioner can practice it in its entirety, or write a treatise to do it complete justice.

Certainly this presentation meets the needs of the majority of the public who think of chiropractic as a musculoskeletal specialty, rather than the portal of entry to the health care system. Everyone should find this an intensely interesting view of a modern contributor to the welfare of the sick and suffering.

The book prepares the prospective patient thoroughly for an encounter with the initial chiropractic examination. The new patient learns the reasons for the various perhaps surprising investigatory procedures which the doctor could not take time to explain in the detail deserved.

The grueling cram course of four years in a chiropractic college provides the education in the biological or basic sciences, the diagnostic skills, and the clinical experience of a general practitioner from any of the schools of generic medicine. The difference is the point of view and methods of patient care. Dr. Dryburgh soon makes the reader aware of the chiropractor's concern for the total person in the maintenance or restoration of the maximum degree of health possible, in contrast to the traditional concentration on the treatment of a disease.

The novice in chiropractic receives a brief and interesting education, while the experienced patient and fellow-practitioner derive insights and explanations to answer many of their asked and unasked questions.

Every reader will be the wiser for having read this book and, I hope, will be prepared to take a greater interest and participation in the maintenance of or return to abundant health.

A. Earl Homewood, D.C.

*SO YOU'RE
THINKING OF GOING TO
A CHIROPRACTOR*

1

The value of being informed

THE body you live in now is the only one you will ever have. When you were conceived, two cells united with a new chromosome pattern from which your body was built. It is a unique structure, with qualities and features that set you apart as an original. No one else in the world is exactly like you.

With care, that body of yours will serve you faithfully and well. It has built into it repairing mechanisms and maintenance features that keep it going through the many health hazards it faces every day. The body has amazing chemical resources, hormones, enzymes and coenzymes, each carrying out its individual function in a delicate but controlled balance.

Every science that studies the body discovers functions, reactions and facilities that astound scientists. They marvel at the body's ability to cope with its changing environment and the incessant and varied demands placed upon it.

What a waste it is to abuse your body! Smokers must be prepared to pay the price for their pleasure; no one doubts now that smoking and cancer are linked. Heavy drinkers and careless drug users are on a dangerous course also; both put their livers under stress. Insurance companies have amassed great folios of information about the hazards of overeating and overweight; every pound of excess fat brings the body nearer to crippling disease and premature death.

Very little is ever said about the abuse of joints and ligaments. We are inclined to take the bone structure of our body for granted. If a joint becomes strained or sprained, we expect it to get better. When the pain is gone, we consider that the problem is past.

Often that is not the end of it, but we prefer to forget the pain and dismiss the problem. We also miss the needed correction that would get rid of the problem for good.

It is quite common for a person whose car is struck from behind in an accident to have a sore neck for a few days and then to have the symptoms fade. The pain goes. There may be a little stiffness or soreness in the

2

neck or between the shoulders, but it is thought to be nothing much; not worth worrying about.

It may be a year or two later that the injured person consults a chiropractor. The major complaint at that time may be headache, shoulder pain, dizziness, recurring nausea, tightness of the upper back muscles or numbness in one or more of the fingers.

The accident may not even be mentioned during the case history until a question brings it to the patient's mind. By this time the chiropractic X-ray will probably show an altered curve on the side view. The normal curve often straightens out where it was originally injured. Damage to ligaments leaves it weak. An irregularity will often be noticed where the ligaments were stretched and the neck has become unstable or movements between vertebrae are irregular or restricted.

A patient came to me this week for treatment for injuries to his neck in an accident three years ago. Palpation of his neck showed that his spine did not move normally where it had been injured. If it is not brought back to nearly normal by chiropractic manipulation, it will become a natural site for future calcium deposits. The body attempts to splint a structurally weak moving part.

Any joint of the body needs to be brought back to its normal range of motion after it is injured, particularly those in the spine. It is important that the joint play be restored as well. These little sideways movements are not part of the major function of a joint, but when they are lost or limited, the joint tends to become a center for discomfort or pain.

As you become informed about chiropractic, you will find it easier to cooperate completely with your

3

chiropractor. You will understand better what is needed to help you get well as quickly as possible. You will know what he is doing, what he expects to be able to accomplish and why he does things in the way that he does.

Dr. Julius Dintenfass writes in the preface of his book *Chiropractic—A Modern Way to Health:* "If you ever become sick, you should know about chiropractic. You should know about this drugless method of healing because it is a different approach which has been winning increasing acceptance—because it is making sick people well. You should know about chiropractic because it may help add years to your life."

Your chiropractor is interested in taking certain measurements of your body and in making specific tests, many of which I shall outline for you. With the resulting information, he will use proven techniques to bring your body parts into a right relationship with each other. They will then be able to function as well as possible without irritating or interfering with one another.

If you drive an automobile when it is out of alignment, parts will wear out quickly. You will be replacing tires in a few thousand miles because the wear is excessive. When parts of the body wear out or are damaged through abuse or misalignment you have a much more serious problem. Some can never be replaced or repaired. If they are removed accidentally or through needed surgery, you can be assured that the replacement parts will not work as well as the originals, or as long.

Every day he practices, your chiropractor fights degeneration of body parts. It is always a pleasure to him to see complete recovery, but he will have his quota

4

of patients who have irreversible conditions. He uses his skills to keep them out of pain, to keep them walking, to keep them from being restricted to wheelchairs. Commit yourself to becoming well informed as to what he is able to do for you so that you do not throw any hurdles in his way in your case.

2

Your chiropractor is an interesting person to know

ONE distinctive aspect of your Doctor of Chiropractic is that he will almost certainly be excited about his profession. So many amazing things happen in his practice that he is stimulated every day.

Advances in the profession have often resulted from studies carried out in offices and clinics around the world. Funds have not been available from governmental and philanthropic bodies for the cross-section of basic chiropractic research and clinical investigation needed, but practitioners have not hesitated to finance their own and university-based research.

The results are often astounding. In Brussels, Belgium, Drs. Henri Gillet and M. Liekens studied the movements of the spine and the unusual movements associated with areas of fixation, and developed a method of finding these areas of trouble. Dr. John L. Faye, of Ottawa, Canada, studied their work and prepared a teaching format to make this research usable in every chiropractic office. Another method of spinal analysis and treatment was devised by Dr. C. S. Gonstead, who discovered and taught the "level disc theory." Drs. W. V. Pierce and Glen Stillwagon of Pennsylvania developed a method of correcting pelvic imbalance and invented a heat-sensing instrument to measure the results of their corrections. Dr. I. N. Toftness, of Cumberland, Wisconsin, originated a light-touch adjustive method and proved its worth by controlled before-and-after X-ray studies, over 5,000 in number, which are available for future research.

These research projects were undertaken by brilliant men and women at their own expense. The whole profession has had the findings made available to it through teaching conferences and seminars, and chiropractic patients around the world have benefited.

Your chiropractor will often mention that he is off to a seminar for a few days. What he is saying is that chiropractic has taken another step forward, and he is keeping up with the advances made in the profession. Chiropractors flock to these teaching conventions. They value both the information they receive and the contact with the thinkers who spearhead the discoveries.

8

Your chiropractor is an interesting person to know

Most chiropractors have an independent spirit. When they chose their career, they knew that they would be depending on their own resources much of the time in caring for the sick and injured, and they were willing to prepare for that responsibility.

Your chiropractor cannot pass the buck to anyone. He carries the weight of your health problem alone. No one stands in the background to protect him or to defend him. He must be well equipped for the task he faces—and he is.

The young men or women entering chiropractic are well aware of the possibility of opposition from the medical people who prescribe drugs in their area. With a comparable length of study, they could be in the allopathic medical profession—that is, with the M.D. degree—where prestige and acceptance are not based on performance alone, but they believe that chiropractic is a valuable alternative and the medical method of choice in many ailments and injuries.

Most people are amazed at the standard of education required to practice chiropractic. The profession has been steadily upgrading for most of this century. To be accepted for enrollment in a chiropractic college a person must have studied at least two years of university-level science. Many applicants have their B.Sc. degree. In a college I visited recently a number of students had obtained their Ph.D. degree before commencing the study of chiropractic.

The four years of chiropractic education are obtained in colleges founded—and maintained and supported—by the profession. The large government grants made to universities, colleges and allopathic medical schools have not yet been available to chiropractic educational institutions, though there may be a change in this policy in the years to come.

During the four years of study your chiropractor covered a wide variety of subjects. He studied anatomy—all body parts including nerves, bones, ligaments, muscles, organs, arteries and veins; physiology—how everything works and the interactions between body parts and substances; embryology—how the body formed from the moment of fertilization until birth; histology—how every tissue cell looks and acts; and pathology—how body tissues and parts degenerate in disease states and ultimately die. He studied biochemistry, microbiology, neurology, public health, hygiene and sanitation, clinical psychology and toxicology—the study of poisonous substances and their effect on the body. He learned how to diagnose ailments and to differentiate among conditions that have many similarities. He covered the subjects of nutrition, rehabilitation and X-ray science and technology.

He became an authority on chiropractic principles and technique and conducted a practice of his own in a teaching outpatient clinic associated with his college before he ever came to your area.

He was allowed to take the examinations of the Board of Examiners only after he had satisfied his alma mater that he had mastered his subjects and had obtained a satisfactory level of excellence in what he had studied. Both written and oral exams still faced him before he could commence his private practice. He is practicing today because he mastered these as well.

In spite of all this preparation, you will occasionally hear someone speak about the chiropractor's limited education. Recently, a member of another health profession in my city spoke of chiropractors taking a "six-month course." It may have been an honest mistake; he probably did not know. Years ago Spencer made the statement: "There is a principle which is a bar against information, which is proof against all argument, and which cannot fail to keep a man in everlasting ignorance. That principle is condemnation before investigation."

Your investigation into chiropractic is a wise action. You will benefit from knowing a science that may bring you more vital health. Your chiropractor is using the principles of chiropractic to correct body function and to resist degenerative changes within you. He strengthens and improves the health of many interrelated tissues and organs by influencing the nerves that govern and control them. While others look for a germ to kill, you and he will be concentrating on building a body that resists invasion and the resulting breakdown.

3

You decided to see a chiropractor

WHEN a patient arrives for his first chiropractic adjustment, he usually feels a little apprehensive. He has never done this before. By the second or third visit this anxiety has usually been dispelled. Your chiropractor understands this tension on your part. He probably feels the same way about visiting his dentist.

Most first-timers know very little about chiropractic, so they make the decision to come on the basis of only a few bits of information.

They usually understand that if any of the twenty-four vertebrae of the spine are in trouble, the chiropractor is the one to see for help. The patient often touches his back and makes the comment: "It feels as though it's pinching right here. I couldn't see how taking a pill would take the pressure off that nerve." His simple logic is more accurate than he realizes.

The new patient is usually an authority on the theme that nerve irritation is painful. Scientific investigation into the mechanisms of pain is extensive, but when a spinal nerve is damaged and begins to swell, he is no longer open to casual discussion about pain. He wants to get rid of it as quickly and as expertly as it can be done.

Those who have inquired further already know that nerve interference in the spine can cause remote symptoms—weakness, degeneration and pain in an organ or tissue far removed from the spine. They come to the chiropractor hoping to find relief from a stomach ulcer, from nausea or dizziness, from monthly menstrual pain or from an asthmatic condition. They want to have the spine checked for any distortions that might be causing or influencing their chronic complaint.

An ever-increasing number of people choose chiropractic because they know a chiropractor will not advise drugs or surgery. They consider chiropractic to be one of the few treatment methods available today with virtually no side effects.

Many patients comment on how relaxed and free-moving they feel after a chiropractic correction to the spine. They had heard about this, but there is often a

14

measure of surprise when they feel it for themselves. Misalignments and fixations in the spine gradually cut back on your range and freedom of movement. Treatment of the spine by your chiropractor is intended to restore this function.

If you were to interview a number of chiropractic patients, you would find that most of them were referred to their chiropractor. Allopathic medical referrals increase as medicine struggles with back pain and distortion, but by far the majority of referrals come from satisfied and healthy chiropractic patients.

The sequence goes like this. A person complains to a friend that he hurts, or that his present therapy is not helping. The friend tells him how chiropractic will help him and urges him to visit his own chiropractor. Some people are slow to respond, but when two or three people point the way to the chiropractor the person in pain makes the move himself or has one of his friends make the appointment for him.

A few weeks later the new patient feels greatly improved and he begins actively sharing with others. The cycle of referring repeats.

Business people facing extreme financial loss by having to go to bed for weeks with back pain search for an alternative approach. Their chiropractor works to keep them on the job while they get better.

You may be one of those people who have heard the words: "Nothing can be done for your spinal condition. You will have to learn to live with it." You now know that everything has not been done that could have been done, if chiropractic has not been explored.

There are lots of people who, on hearing that someone is going for chiropractic help, will immediately say, "Oh! I would never go to a chiropractor." If this happens to you, take a good look at whoever spoke; by rights, he or she should be the healthiest person in the room. Someone opposing any health discipline ought to be in exceptional health, having found a better route to physical wellbeing—but you will be amazed at how many sick and worsening people will want to advise you about your health!

Your decision to benefit from chiropractic correction and care has behind it over eighty-five years of public interaction with this profession. While the public is loud in its appreciation for the relief obtained, statistics have been quietly accumulating. In one study of a thousand herniated and "slipped" discs receiving chiropractic management, the research department of the International Chiropractic Association reported that 96.6 percent of the cases showed improvement, with 49.6 percent achieving complete recovery. These numbers are significant in light of the fact that 82.7 percent of the cases had allopathic medical care before consulting a chiropractor.[1]

The *Journal of the Ohio State Chiropractic Association* reported on a study of 100 children with recurring headaches. After stretching-type treatments, 97 percent of the children never had such headaches again.[2]

Even some members of other health disciplines would agree with your decision to seek chiropractic help. In an article in *The Practitioner*, F. D. Hart, M.D. reported that chiropractic mobilization of the spine resulted in better progress in ankylosing spondylitis (Bechterew's disease) than the use of a corset.[3]

The *Lancet* carried an article prepared by a team of five from the Department of Family and Community

Medicine, University of Utah College of Medicine, entitled "A Comparison of the Effectiveness of Physician and Chiropractic Care," which was the report on a study of workmen's compensation patients. These patients all suffered from back or spinal problems. Of these, 122 were treated by chiropractic methods and 110 were treated using conventional medical approaches. Patients were interviewed to find out how they functioned before and after their accidents and how well they were satisfied with the care they had received. The conclusion was that "the chiropractors appear to have been as effective with the patients they treated as were the physicians." [4]

W. B. Parsons, M.D. wrote an editorial in the *Journal of the College of General Practice of Canada* in which he commented: "When they [physicians] discover the ease with which many conditions that previously they could not relieve respond to manipulation, they almost feel cheated by their medical schools. . . . As for the future, some pessimists feel that the medical profession on this continent has lost by default to the chiropractors and osteopaths its opportunity to serve in this field." [5]

The *Canadian Medical Association Journal* published an explanation by R. A. Leemann, M.D., as follows: "It is increasingly obvious that many painful conditions of the back as well as of more peripheral parts are caused by functional or organic derangements of the spine. With this newer awareness has come improvement in diagnosis and treatment of many painful syndromes. . . . The addition of 'chiropractic' maneuvers to general management permits treatment of the cause rather than the effect." [6]

17

So you're thinking of going to a chiropractor

Your decision to consult a chiropractor may have been made quietly, maybe even with a few misgivings, but the evidence indicates that it was a sound decision, and one from which you are likely to benefit.

Notes

1. Research Department, International Chiropractic Association, Davenport, Iowa. *A Study of 1000 "Herniated and Slipped Discs" Cases Under Chiropractic Care.* n. d.

2. D. Smith, "Neck Stretching Banishes Most Youths' Headaches," *Journal of the Ohio State Chiropractic Association* (April 1971).

3. F. D. Hart, "Treatment of Ankylosing Spondylitis," *The Practitioner* (August 1969).

4. R. L. Kane, C. Leymaster, D. Olsen, F. R. Wooley, F. O. Fisher, "Manipulating the Patient. A Comparison of the Effectiveness of Physician and Chiropractic Care," *Lancet* (June 29, 1974).

5. W. B. Parsons, "Manipulative Medicine, What Is Its Status?" *Journal of the College of General Practice of Canada* (October 1966).

6. R. A. Leemann, *Canadian Medical Association Journal* (April 1958).

4

The case history is your story

ON your first visit to the chiropractor a number of things happened. It is likely that your Doctor of Chiropractic was too busy to explain what he was doing, so I would like to do that for him.

Remember all those questions he asked? They got just a little monotonous, didn't they? He was taking your case history, a vital and important part of your records which he will keep for future reference. Today you are the result of everything that has happened to you through the years.

Injuries of yesterday have left their scars. You may not see the scars, but they are there just the same—in the ligaments, in the muscles, in the joints, and even in the internal organs and their supporting structures.

Athletes provide clear evidence of this, particularly those in contact or collision sports. Football players weave, twist, run at top speed from thrusting starts, crash into each other, fall and squash at the bottom of the pile. Take a look at some of the men who played twenty-five years ago. Unless they took great care to have the damage repaired and the distortions in their joints remedied, they will probably be showing the effect of the earlier damage today and every day.

Some people find the case history tedious. They feel that what troubles them today is important, not the problems of the past.

Many conditions that give trouble today have been sneaking up on you for quite a while. You noticed a little discomfort, leaned away from it, and felt better. Gradually you became conditioned to the minor pain. You got used to it and shrugged it off.

Under questioning you remember that it was there, not just last month, but a year ago—maybe even two or three years ago. Time gets telescoped in our memories.

When you began to be limited by the problem, you made your movements in the direction and to the extent that they were not painful or stiff. Accepting your limitations as normal, you soon began living a life that had boundaries because certain movements hurt. When the questioning involved in taking the case history brings this out, you are surprised and a little annoyed at the discovery.

You may not be aware of the seriousness of some symptoms that you have begun to take for granted. I remember a patient mentioning during his case history that he had once had albumin in the urine while in the army. On occasion he had checked himself for this in the intervening years. It had been positive from time to time for about a year. He was in an advanced stage of a terminal disease, knowing the symptom was there, but treating it casually.

Every variance from the norm is important in a case history. If you notice anything changing, that should be included in your answers. Do you notice tiredness or weakness at a certain time of day? Mention it. Is an act that was easy last year harder to perform now? Tell your chiropractor. Do you find yourself trying to get a deeper breath at times? Have you less appetite or greater thirst? Make sure you tell the whole story. Missing items do not lead to a conclusive diagnosis. Everything is important.

Your chiropractor has studied diseases and the separate changes that take place in your body which lead up to a condition that can be named and identified. Instead of waiting for the full-blown condition to hit you, the chiropractor may be able to spot the early indications and reverse the process by giving the body the ability to fight back. This saves the patient pain and discomfort. As you explain the changes you have noticed, your chiropractor can plan the best course of treatment to bring you back to normal.

Another reason for taking an investigative case history is that a nutritional weakness may show up. A person may casually mention that he bruises easily. He has noticed that bumping the edge of a counter or leaning heavily against a table or desk will often leave a bruise. This may have nothing to do with the condition that brought him to his chiropractor's office, but it does indicate that the patient may need to increase his vitamin C intake to lessen capillary fragility.

A patient may comment, "I often have cramps in my legs. There does not seem to be any reason for this. I'm not working hard." The chiropractor will probably ask a few more questions to see if a calcium deficiency is indicated.

People who have long-term diarrhea or colitis lose quantities of fluid from the system. With the fluid loss there is also a potassium loss which must be made good for normal chemical interchanges in the body to take place.

Your case history begins the moment the chiropractor or his assistant begins filling out your chart. Your age is important. The development and degeneration of certain tissues, as well as variations in hormone activity, are age-linked. Your sex matters because some conditions occur more often in men, other conditions, for example systemic lupus erythematosis, appear more often in women. The length of time you have had the condition often indicates to the chiropractor whether you will achieve full recovery.

As the case history is taken, you will notice that, while you are interested in your chief complaint and how quickly you can be rid of it, your chiropractor is interested in you as a whole person. He knows that a breakdown of tissue or accidental damage to one joint will mean that other parts and tissues are under stress. He will not be satisfied to help one part of your body back to normal health while he ignores another weakened area. If he understands that another problem will develop to the painful stage within a short time, he will want to attend to that need as well as to the obvious and immediate complaint.

You will find that your chiropractor is interested in helping you find the best health you can attain. He is not just a reliever of your pain, although that is extremely important to him.

It is always a point of concern to find how and when the problem began. If healthy tissue is injured by a sudden blow or twist, all the body resources are marshaled to assist in the recovery. When a condition develops slowly over a period of time and gradually becomes bad enough to consult your chiropractor for, the body may have so exhausted its built-in healing mechanisms that it is now ready to adapt to the stubborn problem. Calcium splinting of a weak joint may have begun. There is a great difference in the method of treatment and rate of recovery between the acute accident and the chronic degenerative condition.

I recently examined a woman who had brachial neuritis, a painful condition with nerve interference in the lower neck, and pain in the shoulder and arm radiating down to the hand. X-ray examination showed considerable distortion in the upper cervical spine which I discussed with the patient. She knew of no reason for this but I pointed out that both problems must be treated as one and corrected together.

A short time later the lower neck problem was gone, but the patient was in considerable pain in her upper neck where minimal pain but considerable trouble had been noted. As we probed further, the patient

23

remembered that she had slipped off a swing some time before. The seat had swung back and struck her on the neck, causing the damage. She had completely forgotten the incident.

The upper cervical injuries would have caused later problems. The patient had not sought the help she needed at the time of the accident, but the slow onset of neuritis, from distortion in a nearby spinal area, brought her to my office.

The inquiry into past illnesses is a probe to find if the present acute situation has any relationship to a more prolonged health problem—a link of which the patient is not aware. Questions about illness in blood-family members probe for any factors of heredity in the problem. High blood pressure will sometimes be found in several generations of a family. Some metabolic diseases, such as diabetes, or allergic reactions like eczema, hay fever or hives may be family-linked.

Since the chiropractor will need to decide whether it is safe for you to work or not, be sure that he understands what you do, how you move at work, and what stresses and loads you put on your body, particularly on the weak or injured part. If you were injured on the job, it is absolutely vital that the information available about your injury and the actions involved in it be explained in detail to your chiropractor so that he can accurately report on what you did and what he is doing about it.

Be sure that your chiropractor knows whether you have ever been knocked unconscious, whether you have ever used a cane or crutch, whether you have ever had a bone fracture. He needs to know what other treatment you have had for the condition, particularly what drugs you may be taking at the time of your treatment by him.

Think of your chiropractor as a detective tracking down a criminal—the condition that causes you discomfort. Your chart should contain all the clues you can give to help get the criminal out of your system.

Keep in mind the fact that your chiropractor is just as interested in finding which cases he cannot help as in finding those he can. His success in his profession indicates that he does not disappoint many people. Your case history is one of his chief tools in deciding whether you can get well under chiropractic case management.

Your case history is never complete. When all the information is on file today and the record is finished, the story has not ended. You are still alive. Any change in your condition from day to day is important to keep the chart current. It is your personal story.

5

Insights on your physical examination

 A S your chiropractor stepped into the examining room to give you your physical examination, he knew exactly what he was going to do. With so many items to cover on a new patient, each one of us uses a specific examination procedure to accomplish the task in a reasonable time.

A good percentage of people visiting a chiropractic physician for the first time have already had another kind of treatment for their condition. They have had some form of examination already. To succeed in getting the patient well, the chiropractor must find what others have missed. He must examine carefully what others have passed over casually.

He will first perform a physical examination. Then he will conduct orthopedic, neurological and chiropractic tests, besides examining the spine for evidence of altered relationships between vertebrae, which are responsible for many of the relevant signs he discovers.

The physical examination is conducted by using sight, touch and instrumental checking. From the first moment he is watching for any departure from the norm. He will note how you stand, sit, shake hands and talk. Any jerky or clumsy movements will be recorded.

He knows about your pain from the history you communicated. He will watch to see how the pain is affecting you. Many people become depressed by pain that continues for a long time. The malingerer wears it like a badge. Others become agitated by it, or develop manic evidences. The stress of pain, when the patient has borne it well, will sometimes show in the eyes, in the speech pattern or in the breathing. Though your chiropractor is not just a "pain doctor," you can be sure that all through the examination his first goal is the elimination of your pain.

From your own observation you will recognize a number of different gaits. The stroke victim drags the partially paralyzed leg. The person who bends forward from the waist and takes a number of tiny steps to start may suffer from Parkinson's disease. A person with multiple sclerosis usually has a stiff walk that is best described as choppy. If cerebellar disease is present, a person may walk as though he is drunk.

Most physical signs are as easy to log as these irregularities in gait. You just need to know what you are looking for, and what it means when you find it.

The examination of the head and neck is based on checking all the normal findings and listing the unusual for a later recheck. Even the symptoms your chiropractor will not treat will act as a guide as to how your body is functioning. On a later examination, improvement may indicate that your body is better able to handle its problems, probably as a result of the chiropractic care you sought.

Your chiropractor is interested if your ears are full of wax, but he is just as concerned if you hold your head so that one ear is usually higher than the other. Since the first chiropractic patient claimed great improvement of a hearing impairment, you may be shown how to check any hearing limitation you may have, to detect at home if the keenness of your hearing improves.

As he looks through the pupil of the eye with his ophthalmoscope, the chiropractic practitioner is concerned particularly with the area where the optic nerve, the nerve of sight, enters the eye. He has an indication here of how quickly you are aging. If the blood vessels cause dents in one another where they cross, you are losing some of the elasticity so essential to youthfulness.

In headache cases, he will inspect the same area of the eye to see if there are any evidences of pressure behind the eye, pushing the tissue slightly forward. He is checking out the possibility of a brain tumor or any other space-occupying lesion.

He will also check for eye movement to be sure

29

that the third, fourth and sixth cranial nerves are well and functioning.

In fact, since he is a chiropractor, concerned about nerve response and function, he will be likely to check all the cranial nerves. These twelve nerves come out of the skull through a variety of openings and are vitally important to our health.

The first cranial nerve carries our sense of smell, the second our sense of sight. The third, fourth and sixth control our eye movements. The fifth powers the muscles we chew with and carries the sensation from the skin of the face. The seventh innervates the muscles of facial expression and is the nerve involved in the facial paralysis of Bell's palsy. The eighth cranial nerve enables us to hear and to maintain balance. The ninth has to do with taste and the protective gag reflex. The tenth is called the vagus nerve. It is wide-ranging and has to do with many of the automatic actions of the heart, lungs and abdominal organs; it is tested by swallowing. The eleventh cranial nerve controls the trapezius muscle and is tested by shrugging. The twelfth cranial nerve controls the actions of the tongue and is tested by sticking out the tongue. The patient is often unaware that the cranial nerves are being checked.

Some people are surprised when the chiropractor takes their blood pressure, listens to their heart, records their pulse rate, weight and height. As your chiropractor checks your abdomen and other areas of your body for masses or swelling, or your ankles to see if they pit from water retention in the tissues, remember that he is not treating a disease entity but a person, a whole person, with a number of varied health needs. He needs to know everything he can learn about that person. Besides,

30

it is good for his ego to be able to check later the degree of health improvement he has brought into your life!

The urine examination is often thought to be a hospital or lab routine, but in many chiropractic offices it is part of the initial physical examination. The urine contains vital information about the metabolism of the body. It often gives the first clear sign of a degenerative condition. Normal urine when first collected is slightly acid, with a pH of about 6. If a specimen is found to be highly alkaline, we suspect the patient of indulging in alkalizers or using bicarbonate of soda. A highly acid urine is found in a number of serious conditions: diabetes mellitus, gout, chronic nephritis, leukemia, acute articular rheumatism or scurvy.

The presence of protein in the urine (albuminuria) may be associated with serious kidney infections, tuberculosis, inflammation of the kidney pelvis, diabetes mellitus, lupus erythematosis and other degenerative diseases.

When sugar or glucose is consistently found in the urine, the culprit is usually diabetes mellitus. It is also present in a number of other conditions such as increased intracranial pressure, chronic liver disease, hyperactive pituitary or thyroid glands and sometimes in pregnancy or during emotional upheavals.

Bilirubin comes from destroyed red blood cells. When bilirubin breaks down in large amounts, a substance called urobilin will be found in the urine. This indicates serious conditions like hemolytic jaundice or pernicious anemia. Urobilin levels may also be high in infectious hepatitis, congestive heart failure, malaria, lobar pneumonia and pregnancy.

If urobilin and urobilinogen are found together

31

in the urine, and there is no hemolytic anemia in the body, then the liver is either infected seriously or malfunctioning.

Urobilinogen alone indicates hemolytic anemias with their increase in dead red blood cells, liver damage with an upset in the secretion through the bile duct, or serious infections in the body, with massive red blood cell destruction.

The kidney is a wonderful filter, processing 180 liters of plasma-like substance called filtrate each and every day. This is four and a half times as much fluid as there is in the entire body. Of this large quantity only about a liter is passed out of the body as urine. The rest is put back into the general circulation while the impurities filtered out pass from the body in the urine. Blood found in the urine is a sign of trouble. A kidney stone may have cut the inside of the urinary passage and the bleeding takes place beyond reach of the filtering action; often, blood in the urine is the result of damage in the ureters, bladder or urethra, or of serious inflammation or infection.

The urine analysis adds considerable information to the physical examination and gives conclusive diagnostic authority in the areas it covers. Never hesitate to get the specimen to your chiropractor when he requests it.

6

Orthopedic tests commonly used in chiropractic examination

THE next step in chiropractic investigation involves the use of a number of tests and procedures developed through the years by researchers in many countries. As they painstakingly repeated tests on various members and tissues of the body, a scale of normal responses was developed. Gradually variations from the norm were linked with specific problems, because they consistently turned up when those problems were present.

Once this was known, the tests were organized in such a way that a number of them could be performed quickly yet accurately on every patient. Their results are a consistent aid to the diagnosis of chiropractic problems.

It is likely that you were given twenty-five or more tests when you first visited your chiropractor, and that a number of these were repeated from time to time to monitor your progress. The order of the tests and examination procedures outlined for your information varies with different chiropractors; the gathering of the information is the vital thing. Some of the neurological tests will be mentioned in the chapter dealing with a chiropractor's daily experience.

Keep in mind that these tests can be performed by the layman as well as the professional. The body will yield its information to anyone if the test is accurately performed. Correcting the distortion that gives a positive sign in any of the tests is work for the professional. If you discover a problem, be sure to leave the treatment of it to your chiropractor.

Normal range of motion for the cervical spine is well established. While sitting erect you should be able to tilt your head forward about 60°, backward 30°, to each side about 40°, and to rotate it without tilting about 60°—all these without straining. Testing the range of motion often uncovers a gradual loss of mobility of which the patient is unaware. It is not unusual for a patient under chiropractic treatment to remark how good it is to be able to look over the shoulder while backing up in an automobile.

The lower back can be tested for range of motion

in a similar manner. Forward bending should reach close to 90°. Backward bending should be 30°. Lateral tilting from the waist will be 25° to 35° both ways. Twisting from the waist should be about 30°. Athletes will chuckle at these norms, but they will apply to most of us. Lower back range of motion should be checked with care if the lumbar spine is painful. Do not push past the point where pain wants to stop the movement.

You should be able to move your shoulder 170°. Starting with your arm at the side, you should be able to bring it above your head, without bending the elbow, to within 10° of perpendicular. This applies to both sideward and forward movements.

If you lie on your back on the floor with your upper arm stretched away from the body and your lower arm perpendicular to the floor, you should be able to move your hand downward 90° in either direction, so that both the palm and the back of your hand can hit the floor. Normal shoulder movement allows you to lie face down on the floor with your arm at your side, close to the body, and to move it backward 30° without bending the elbow. Your elbow, when it is used like a hinge, should move 150° in its arc of motion.

With your elbow still, your hand should be able to turn 180° from palm down to palm up for normal range of motion. Your wrist should have 90° of motion palmward and 70° of motion backward.

Your hip should flex 110° forward and 30° backward. If you lie on your back and raise one leg out of the way, the other hip should let the leg swing outward 50° and past the midline 30°.

Your chiropractor may not check all these ranges

35

of motion. He will normally check any joints having problems, as well as the spine.

The Trendelenberg test, conducted while you are still standing, is performed by having you raise one leg to hip level with the knee bent. The buttock on the same side should lift up. If it lowers, or even stays at the same height when the leg lifts, gluteal weakness is present; this may be due to a number of reasons, some of them serious.

Sacroiliac fixation—loss of flexibility—can be very painful. You can check for its presence in someone by having him walk in place while you place a finger on his sacrum about two inches below the beltline close to the center and the next finger about three inches to the side. As the person walks, you feel definite movement in each of the locations if there is no fixation. The inflexibility of fixation makes the back more liable to needless future injury.

A patient cannot walk on the toes in the case of many injuries to the fifth lumbar nerve root. Heel walking difficulty points to either the fourth or the fifth lumbar nerve root.

The diagnostic indication called Kemp's sign is found by having the patient bend backwards while he also twists and leans to one side. He then takes the same obliquely backward twist to the other side. The sign is positive when he feels pain down the side toward which he bends. He may have lateral disc protrusion, other disc involvement, degenerative joint disease, or a problem with a vertebra.

For low back pain, a number of tests help to pinpoint where the problem is and to indicate the degree of seriousness. Lasegue's test is a standard one and is done

36

with the patient lying face up on the examining table. With one hand the chiropractor prevents the knee from bending; with the other, he lifts the heel from the table until the leg is perpendicular. If a severe lumbosacral distortion, fifth lumbar disc damage, or lower lumbar intervertebral foramen occlusion is present, the leg will not lift, while held straight, to the 90° position; it may lift only 30° or 50°. Usually, one leg will lift further than the other. Severe sacroiliac injury will also limit the Lasegue test.

When the Lasegue test is positive, it is usually followed immediately by the Braggard test. The leg is lowered from the point where it caused pain to the level where it is barely comfortable. The chiropractor then pushes the ball of the foot toward the knee. If this test is positive, the pain returns. Positive Braggard indicates spinal nerve root irritation and may point to the need to investigate for disc herniations or sciatica. If the good leg is raised and the painful leg has increased pain, this is a positive Fajersztajn sign and indicates that a space-occupying lesion may be present.

In low back injury the pain is often thought to be in the hip as well. A simple test to clear up concern over hip joint involvement was designed by a researcher named Patrick and is called the Fabere-Patrick test. The first part of the name is made up from the movements the hip is put through—*f*lexion, *ab*duction, *e*xternal *r*otation and *e*xtension. This test is done by putting the ankle of one foot over the opposite knee and pushing down on the bent knee until the leg is parallel with the top of the examining table. If the hip is diseased, this test will be exceptionally painful—even impossible.

When the forgoing tests suggest that a lumbosacral disc may be defective or that a lumbosacral distortion or sacroiliac damage is present, Lewin's test will help confirm the diagnosis. The patient stands erect and straightens the knees to the limit. If they snap back into a more relaxed position or if the straightening of the leg is painful, the test is positive.

Some difficulty exists in differentiating between lumbosacral pain and pain which originates in the sacroiliac joint. Goldthwaite's test helps to tell them apart. The examiner places his hand beneath the fifth lumbar vertebra with the patient lying on his back. He then asks the patient to lift the painful leg while giving any needed assistance. As the patient lifts his straight leg, the examiner feels for the beginning of movement at the fifth lumbar level. If the patient's pain begins before movement commences in the spine, the problem is probably linked with the sacroiliac area. If the spine moves before the pain begins, the source of pain is usually located in the lower lumbar spine or in the lumbosacral disc area.

The Soto-Hall test also helps to locate the level of injury. With the patient lying face up on the examining table, the examiner puts one hand under the patient's head and the other on the sternum. He lifts the head while putting mild pressure on the sternum. This gradually tightens the posterior spinal ligaments. When the tightening reaches the level of the involved vertebra, the patient will feel discomfort or pain at that level of the spine.

Immediately following the Soto-Hall test, your chiropractor may have asked you to move higher on the table so that your head extended over its end. If he then tipped your head backwards and turned it to one side for over half a minute and repeated this procedure on the other side, he was testing your vertebral arteries. This is called Houle's test by some practitioners and Wallenberg's test by others. If you experience vertigo during the test, you may have narrowing or kinking of the vertebral artery on the side on which testing causes the vertigo.

In low back problems a number of tests to differentiate a sacroiliac problem from lumbar or lumbosacral distortion are performed with the patient lying face down.

First, lift the foot on the side of involvement so that the knee flexes 90° or more. If pain radiates to the lumbosacral area or to the sacroiliac after you pass 90°, the test is positive for the area that hurts.

Then flex the heel to the buttocks on the same side, lifting the thigh off the examining table. This is called Yeoman's test. Positive findings on this test indicate that the third and fourth intervertebral discs should be carefully investigated. If the thigh must be raised from the table for the heel to touch the buttocks, the problem may be in the fifth lumbar intervertebral disc area.

Ely's test is similar except that the heel is touched to the buttock on the opposite side. Pain in this test points to the sacroiliac.

These tests are performed, one after the other, so quickly and smoothly by your chiropractor that you hardly realize how thorough the examination has been until you go over the findings with him. The tests follow each other in a plan that gives the patient as little inconvenience and discomfort as possible.

This sampling of the tests your chiropractor uses

will help you to understand what he is doing as he examines and reexamines. Every patient recovers at his own rate. It is important for your chiropractor at any time to know the amount of correction you have attained and what percentage of total response can be conservatively expected for you.

Be careful, if you are given any of the tests outlined, that you use very little force in any direction. Do not try to make a test appear normal. The limitations you discover, if any, should warn you that trouble exists which requires help.

The body has a phenomenal ability to return to normal with proper care and treatment. The orthopedic tests are a great help in initially finding the source of your problem. The chiropractic approach is to correct the problem at the source rather than doctoring the symptoms. As you improve, you will have fewer positive results in your orthopedic examination. This enables your chiropractor to chart accurately your return to normal health.

7

Chiropractic neurological procedures

Y OUR nerves form a complete net-work of control. Every part of your body receives tiny nerve filaments which tell it what to do. If you could remove all the tissues from a body but nerves, a perfect body likeness would be left, made up of the threadlike nerves which compose your nervous system.

Every artery is surrounded by nerves. Every muscle cell has an activating nerve.

Every organ in the body has nerves to stimulate it, nerves to slow it down and nerves to control the functions of its cells.

The nervous system is like a switchboard connecting the cells of the brain to those of the tissues and organs. If a controlling nerve center in the brain is damaged, the organs or tissues served by that nerve cannot function properly.

You have often seen this in stroke patients. Blood leaks out of a capillary in the brain, and a number of motor or action cells are damaged. Immediately, the muscles served by that area of the brain are paralyzed. The future usefulness of the arm or leg involved depends on how completely the brain heals. There is nothing wrong with the muscle cells in the injured limb, but if the brain cells are dead the paralysis is permanent.

The same kind of paralysis results when the nerve that connects the brain cells to the tissue cells is damaged. In auto accidents the spinal cord is sometimes severed. Everything below the level of damage is suddenly paralyzed, never to move of its own volition again. The brain cells may be healthy and the tissue cells may be healthy, but the connecting nerve pathway has been interrupted.

Each nerve is a bundle of many hundreds of nerve cells (neurons), which transmit electrochemical impulses along their fibers (axons), which may be up to three feet in length. The motor neurons, arising in the brain, join to form the motor nerves, which are channeled into the spinal column, then spread out once more through the openings between the vertebrae to control every part of the body.

Sensory neurons, originating in all body parts, form the sensory nerves, transmitting information to the brain, once again joining together to pass through the spinal column.

The neurons running between the brain and the spinal column are referred to as the upper neurons; those connecting the spinal cord and body parts are the lower neurons.

The brain is in control of the body through this vast network of fibers. It knows what is happening at every level and provides everything that is needed to make it happen.

If the brain decides to lift an arm, the impulse travels down the spine to the lower cervical region, and the impulse passes to the muscle cells that must contract to do this. At the same time, the muscle cells that oppose this action are informed that they should lessen their tone. The blood supply to the shoulder and elbow will increase slightly to provide the metabolic energy required. The muscles supporting the shoulder will also increase their tone slightly, so that the action will not twist the rest of the body. The control is balanced and complete.

Your chiropractor is not involved with brain cell damage or with the severance of the spinal cord. He is concerned with interference with the nerve fibers on their route from brain cell to tissue cell and from tissue cell back to the brain again.

The place of greatest hazard to the nerve is the opening through which it emerges from the spine. At this point it leaves the protection of the spinal column and makes its way through the tissues to its destination.

Such an opening is called an intervertebral foramen; these openings exist between the vertebrae all the way

43

down the spine. The intervertebral foramina are not simply openings in the bone with solid protective boundaries. The upper part of each is formed by a notch in the vertebra above, and the lower part by a notch in the vertebra below.

If the vertebrae of the spine get out of alignment with each other, the notches no longer match perfectly and the contents of the opening are pushed together.

An artery, veins, a lymph vessel, a small nerve and the large spinal nerve all pass through this small opening. When they are compressed, nerve interference takes place which will affect the body in two definite ways: the sensory message to the spinal cord and the brain will be influenced by the interference, and the reverse traffic of nerve impulses to the tissues will be affected.

Your chiropractor examines the nervous system to be sure that the nerves involved can be restored to health.

He taps the tendon between the kneecap and the shin with his reflex hammer. The sudden stretch of the muscle sends a message to the brain. As the impulse reaches the end of the first neuron and skips across to the second nerve cell in the spinal cord which goes right to the brain, it also sends an impulse to the motor nerve at its own level telling it to get the leg out of danger.

The normal response is a gentle kick as the muscles start to contract and then the defensive action is called off by the brain as unnecessary.

If the lower neurons are severely damaged or cut, there will be no kick. The message does not get around to the spinal cord and back. The circuit is broken.

If the upper neurons are severely damaged or cut, the kick will be very strong. The message does get

44

around to the spinal cord and back to the muscle, but there is no overriding control from the brain. The message never reaches the brain. The route of travel is damaged so that the impulses cannot pass through.

The reflex arcs of a number of spinal segments are easy to test with the reflex hammer, a tool specially made for testing. If the patellar reflex which we have been discussing is normal, it indicates that the fourth lumbar nerve on the side being tested is intact. The Achilles reflex, tested by tapping the Achilles tendon while the patient kneels on a chair or table, tests the reflex arc through the first sacral nerve.

The biceps reflex, tested by tapping the tendon of the biceps, just in front of the elbow hinge, tests the integrity of the fifth cervical nerve. A gentle examiner always puts his finger over the biceps tendon and communicates the tap through his own finger. The sixth cervical nerve is tested by tapping the tendon of the brachioradialis muscle. This is about an inch above the wrist, slightly around toward the back of the arm from the base of the thumb. The seventh cervical nerve can be tested by tapping the tendon of the triceps, behind the elbow.

When brain damage is suspected for any reason, or when any upper motor neuron damage is possible, the Babinski test is often used as a first indicator. This is the test in which the chiropractor strokes the sole of your foot with a sharp instrument to see if you curl your toes downward. Be glad if you do. The injured person points his big toe upward and spreads the other four open while pointing them downward. To perform this test the stroke must be done up the outside of the sole of the foot and across the ball of the foot from the

45

side of the little toe to the great toe. Newborn babies give a positive result on this test for a short time but it is not indicative of pathology in them.

A similar response in the toes was evoked by Chaddock's test, which is easily performed by stroking a prominence of the bone above the ankle on the outside of the leg. This will reinforce the Babinski findings.

Every reflex arc has in it a number of component parts. The stimulus is received by an end organ specifically prepared to receive a certain type of sensation. The sensory neuron picks up the impulse and takes it to the spine. A linking neuron takes the impulse from the back of the spinal cord where it enters to the front of the cord. The motor neuron leaves the front of the spinal cord and goes to the muscle or other tissue that needs to be stimulated.

The chiropractor uses a pin or a pinwheel to test various areas of skin if he suspects that some sensation is being blocked. By plotting the area of numbness, he is able to discover which spinal segments are involved. This is a help to him in his chiropractic examination of the spine. The areas of the body served by each nerve root have been clearly located, so the pinwheel examination is very exact.

You may have wondered why your chiropractor asked you to stand still with your eyes closed for a few moments. He does this if he feels your coordination is affected and you may have a cerebellar lesion; it is called the Romberg test. If he asked you to keep your eyes closed and touch your forefingers in front of you, or touch your finger to your nose, or your heel to your skin, he was checking areas deep in your nervous system of vital importance to you. Your chiropractor is interested in the whole person. He looks beneath the surface.

46

8

The chiropractic use of x-rays

YOU were probably surprised when your chiropractor invited you to look over your X-ray pictures with him. It is almost standard procedure for chiropractors and their patients to go over the films together, noting the distortion pattern, considering the thickness and shape of disc spaces and assessing the phase of degeneration that may be present.

Some people are shocked to realize

that these black-and-white shadows are so revealing. They find it hard to believe that, without any previous preparation, they are able to see for themselves the tilting or rotation of vertebrae, the formation of arthritic spurs, or the difference caused by a twist in the pelvis in shape and appearance of body parts normally identical.

The chiropractor usually studies the body as it is in action. That is why he often has the patient stand erect for X-ray examination. The weight and stress of standing is then on the body framework, and areas of distortion and trouble show more clearly than when one is at rest. These are further emphasized as the chiropractor marks and measures the parts under study.

In many chiropractic offices the films are automatically processed and available to the chiropractor within five minutes. He is able to see them almost at once, but may not go over them with the patient until he has gathered all the information about the person. He may even want to do a number of test adjustments before reviewing all the findings. You may be sure, however, that he knows very quickly what the X-ray films show.

The X-ray pictures are to a chiropractor what a blueprint is to a architect or engineer. The location of body parts is well established by the anatomy texts. Your personal pictures are compared with known norms to find where and why you differ. Correction is always planned to bring you back as close to normal as possible.

Your chiropractor knows how to get a maximum of information from a minimum number of views. He measures small relationships between vertebrae to locate possible sites of nerve irritation. He compares the millimeters of rotation of bones in the spine against one

48

another. He looks for tilting and wedging, items of little importance to those who are interested only in fractures, dislocations and pathology. He measures individual vertebrae for rotation, tilting, forward or backward placement and for improper spacing of any kind. He is looking for evidence of disc damage, degeneration of the bone or disc and for any encroachment involving the spinal nerves that might cause nerve interference.

He is also able to calculate the degree of pelvic twisting, if any, by measuring and comparing the openings of the pelvis as outlined on the films. Deviations from the normal position of pelvic balance are also indicated to him by the comparative locations of a number of pelvic landmarks.

One of the pleasing things about chiropractic is that the chiropractor is able to show his patient the problem that he is treating, and is able to explain what he expects to accomplish. Situations in the spine that may be irreversible will also be evident, so that the patient can know exactly what to anticipate.

The chiropractic X-ray examination is a very important piece of evidence for the patient's file. It is often the basis of the final decision as to whether the patient will be accepted for treatment or not. If contraindications are found in the orthopedic, neurological or chiropractic examinations, the X-ray will provide the needed information to put the final piece in the puzzle.

The use of the Roentgen ray was discovered in 1895, the year chiropractic was first practiced. It is a diagnostic tool of great value. Instead of looking at the patient and probing from the outside, the chiropractor is able to look *through* the patient and see the body parts superimposed on each other in a shadowgraph effect.

49

Since bone is the densest tissue, it stands out most clearly. The chiropractor is able to see the bones in their actual, not just their theoretical, relationships to each other. Bony abnormalities need never be dealt with at the guessing level. Their presence is clearly evident in the group of X-ray pictures.

One of the greatest values of the chiropractic X-ray is that it enables the chiropractor to eliminate from his practice those conditions which he does not wish to treat. A person with multiple myeloma can be detected by X-ray examination even if he should pass all other tests. If a bone or part of a bone is missing or indistinct on the film, further investigation will sometimes indicate malignant destruction of the bone tissue. Fractures and dislocations also sometimes appear on chiropractic X-ray pictures and the patient may be referred for surgical repair.

Chiropractic was the first health profession to set up a National Quality Assurance and Radiation Safety Program to control the professional use of examination by X-ray. This program, in effect throughout the United States of America, was established through chiropractic's Federation of State Licensing Boards.

Collimators are now standard equipment on chiropractic X-ray installations. The purpose of the collimator is to limit the area of exposure of any patient to the size of the film in the unit at the time the X-ray examination is made. Most rays outside of the part of the body being examined are absorbed by the filters and lead shields in the collimator, eliminating unnecessary primary and secondary radiation.

Collimators are now mandatory in many areas, but chiropractors were equipping their X-ray units with

50

them long before the law required their use simply because they are a part of high-quality radiographic technique.

Chiropractors almost never take full body X-ray pictures, but do use full spine X-rays frequently. This gives a view of all of the spinal vertebrae on a single film about three feet long. The full spine chiropractic postural X-ray picture gives an indication of the body's ability to cope with the internal distortion of the patient's spine.

If the sacrum is lower on one side than the other, the vertebra immediately above it will tilt. If all of the vertebrae maintained this tilt, the body would lean markedly to one side and the head would be carried in a most unusual position, off to the side. Internal body mechanisms try to put the head directly over the center of balance in the pelvis. Subluxated vertebrae have lost the normal relationship to the vertebrae above or below them on the spinal column. This often disturbs the balance. A plumb line dropped from the center of balance in the upper cervical vertebrae will often miss the pelvic center of balance by half an inch. This places strain on many areas and creates functional twists and curves in the spine. Curvatures of the spine are well known. Full spine X-ray views make this kind of measuring possible and eliminate the risk of missing this important diagnostic information.

51

9

The chiropractic examination

WHEN all the information has been gathered by physical examination, neurological probing, orthopedic testing and X-ray analysis, there still remains that part of the examination that puts it all together. Planning the treatment will also require the findings of the chiropractic examination.

This is where the chiropractor's eyes and fingers pick up the pieces of information that are unique to chiropractic. When this knowledge is added to the data already on your chart, your chiropractor will be able to plan the treatment you require.

Your chiropractor is concerned with the maintenance and restoration of normal function. He does this through the adjustment of the still and moving relationships between bones of the body. He assists this correction and stabilizes it by any necessary adjustment in the holding elements of body joints. He confirms his findings and his progress in treatment by checking the body balance from time to time with techniques that have long been part of chiropractic.

That is why you will notice him looking at you carefully at times. He wants to know which ear is higher, which way your head inclines and the degree of turn with which you carry it when you are relaxed. The comparative levels of shoulders, hips, and the angle of your waistline are significant to him. He will note quickly whether your indentation at the waist is flatter on one side than on the other. As he touches you, he will be comparing the levels on each side of landmarks like the posterior superior iliac spine (PSIS).

If one PSIS is higher than the other when you are standing and the opposite PSIS is higher when you lie face down, you have a spinal problem.

As you lie face down, your chiropractor will check to see if one ankle is higher than the other. Tight muscles or damaged ligaments in the pelvis or upper leg will sometimes give the appearance of a short leg. As he flexes the knees and checks leg length with the knees bent, he gains more information about pelvic imbalance.

He may move various joints very slightly, particu-

54

larly in the area of injury. He is checking for joint play, that elusive extra function of a joint so often lost in injuries. If joint play is not restored as healing takes place, the injured part becomes a potential site for future pain or degenerative changes.

The chiropractic touching examination of the spine is called spinal palpation. To learn the art of palpation, the chiropractic student does everything possible to increase the sensitivity of his fingertips. I remember how we struggled in undergraduate days to locate human hair and chart its location beneath ten sheets of note paper, so that our fingers would become sensitive to the tissues beneath the skin.

This sense of touch becomes keenly developed and is valuable to you as your chiropractor runs his fingers along your spine, searching for clues. It is not unusual for the patient to express surprise when the chiropractor puts his hand on the focus of pain almost as soon as he touches the spine. He is not necessarily feeling spinal distortion; the actual derangement of bone may be minimal, and it is often the subtle changes in the tissues around the subluxation or fixation that he recognizes.

When a spinal nerve is irritated for any reason, tissues at that level go through a process of change. The irritated nerve tightens up the tissues, increasing their tone. They feel firmer and more highly tensed than is normal. This tension may come and go as the body struggles to restore the status quo. Throughout this period palpation will almost always show indications of subtle changes in the spinal tissues. Eventually the chronic problem leaves an area of weakness where tissues have a permanent variance from the norm.

The pioneers in chiropractic were often strong,

dynamic personalities. When someone would ask how they found these troubled areas with such apparent ease, they would joke that they had X-rays in their fingertips. What they were really saying was that they had learned the art of detecting underlying changes in spinal tissues. They had developed the ability to tell where the problems were located.

Three indications of trouble that are always significant in the spinal examination are tenderness on pressure, edema or swelling, and spasm in the muscles associated with the vertebrae.

As a result of a study in Belgium headed by Dr. Henri Gillet, an important dimension has been added to chiropractic palpation. Methods, standards and comparison techniques have been prepared to find and record abnormal movement between vertebrae, detectable while the spine is in motion.

When the moving spine is palpated using the methods developed by this research, areas of altered or restricted movement are located and can later be accurately rechecked to determine the progress made by the chiropractic correction.

Your chiropractor also has an approach to muscle examination that enables him to determine if the muscles in the area of spinal subluxation have been weakened. Testing individual muscles for weakness is exacting but accurate. This dimension of examining provides one more approach to calculating the total benefits received while the treatment is in progress.

10

How to help your chiropractor help you

BEFORE you undertake a course of chiropractic adjustments, certain things should be clear to you. If they are, your relationship with your chiropractor and your personal benefits from chiropractic can be enhanced.

First of all, be sure you understand what the findings indicate for you and what the chiropractic physician expects to be able to accomplish for you. It is important that you know where you are going so that you do not feel disappointed when you get there.

No promises of miracle cures should be expected, nor are they likely to be given. You need to know what is involved in the planned program of care ahead of you and whether it will lead to normal or near-normal function. If there is the probability or possibility of permanent handicap or disability, you should prepare for that eventuality.

Some patients are impatient to get started and do not listen well as their chiropractor reports his findings. Your chiropractor will want to make his explanation as clear as possible. Make sure you understand him, so that you know what he plans to do.

Be sure that you understand the three phases of chiropractic treatment and recovery. Your chiropractor is not a "pain doctor," interested only in relieving your painful symptoms. He is interested in getting you well, so that he will not see you a few years later with degenerative processes working in your spine which could have been avoided with care at the time of first injury.

The acute phase of your problem is the period of pain or other severe symptoms. You are very aware of your problem because of the symptoms it presents. Your chiropractor will do everything in his power to get you out of this pain. He will not mask it with drugs, but he will help the body correct the cause of the pain. Many problems exist in the body before the painful stage is reached. These will still need to be corrected, but termination of the painful period is sweet relief.

Once the pain is minimized or gone, the corrective phase of chiropractic adjusting begins. This is the rebuilding period. The distortion or fixation in the spine that brought the discomfort is gradually adjusted so that normal function will be regained and the cause of the problem removed. Points of nerve interference that could trigger the painful situation again are manipulated and strengthened. Degenerative processes already in action are brought under control if possible. Treatment is administered to slow down the degeneration of tissues, stop it, or even reverse it if it has not gone too far.

Correction is carried to the limit of your body's ability to respond. Then the sustaining phase of treatment begins. You will be checked on a regular basis for signs of any further degenerative changes in the spine so they may be stopped before they become a problem. When the spine is checked, adjustments are made to stabilize and strengthen any of the previously weakened areas and to prevent the development of fixations near the site of previous injury.

This is the kind of care we give our automobiles. We do not usually treat our bodies like this until breakdown in some part has begun and has given us a warning. Patients who discipline themselves to follow instructions faithfully during the sustaining phase of treatment have a good possibility of avoiding further spinal distress. Health in organs and tissues throughout the body can also be enhanced by the balance and functional integrity that results from spinal care on a regular basis.

This sustaining treatment of your spine enables your chiropractor to keep it from deteriorating and repeating the pattern of distortion and pain that brought you to his office in the first place.

Be sure that you understand sufficiently what is being done for you so that you can commit yourself to

59

carry through until the job is done. Just as a bricklayer hates to leave a wall half built, your chiropractor hates to leave a spine pain-free but in trouble. The patient who fails to complete his treatment often walks around with a slowly degenerating spine, saying, "I feel fine!"

What he should really be saying is, "I don't feel any back pain—yet." His tomorrows will likely have pain in them, pain that could have been avoided with a minimum of care.

An uncle of mine is a chiropractor. While I was establishing practice as a new graduate, I assisted in his clinic, which was staffed by several chiropractors. I heard him say over and over to new patients as he outlined the treatment they needed, "Please do not take the first adjustment in this clinic unless you plan to take the last one." He knew that it would take a certain length of time to obtain the needed correction, and that the patient had to commit himself to that time in order to avoid disappointment.

During the adjustment it is important that you avoid stress or tension. Leave yourself enough time so that you can wait a few minutes while your chiropractor finishes his work on the patient preceding you. Chiropractors are not time-wasters, but they will not hurry. It takes time to do the necessary rechecks and give an accurate adjustment. He will not rush with you, either, and you know how important that is to you.

Practice relaxing while you are on the treatment table. Remember that you and your chiropractor are on the same team, working for your complete recovery. A relaxed patient is much easier to adjust. It takes less force to move a vertebra in a relaxed, limp patient. You will feel the adjustment less if you just let go.

60

Do not try to help, either. Let your chiropractor do his work. In adjusting, the placement of the arms and legs must often be exact for the best results. Every body angle becomes important. Your chiropractor knows what to do. Let him do it!

After the adjustment, you should avoid strenuous activity for at least an hour. Remember, bones do not "click" in and out of place. The sound you sometimes hear is a vacuum pop comparable to the crack you can make with your knuckles.

The chiropractic adjustment aims to accomplish three things: realign the vertebrae; slightly open the disc space; and restore fixation between vertebrae to normal movement. This is done basically to free the spinal nerves from any interference.

Heavy lifting, twisting, or excessive reaching or stretching may put enough opposing stress on the vertebrae involved so that some of the correction is lost. Recovery takes longer if you do this very often.

Do not expect miracle cures! In some acute situations the patient will obtain immediate relief from the pain, but usually improvement is gradual. The time period between headaches gets longer. You gradually feel movement coming back to normal in an injured shoulder. The knifelike pains in your low back begin to lose their edge. Your stomach ulcer begins to lose its bite. These are the usual signs that you are getting better under chiropractic care.

After the adjustment, follow your chiropractor's instructions. Do exactly as he says. If he advises you to use heat in a certain place for a certain length of time, use it! If he gives you a timetable for ice application, follow it! If he wants you to wear a cervical collar, wear

61

it! Some patients expect their chiropractor to do it all, and often he does. Your total cooperation is essential for best and lasting results.

When the pain is gone, you have reached the place where many people experience a reinjury. There is not too much danger of overextending yourself during the acute and painful period following an injury. You are careful; every move is calculated because you do not want to aggravate an already painful part. As soon as the pain leaves, you want to make up for lost time. You are sure that you can pick up that outboard motor or pull out the sofa to clean behind it.

The pain returns immediately. Your thinking goes in one of two directions, depending on your personality.

"That chiropractor didn't help me!" That's unreasonable, but it often happens. People find it easier to blame another. It makes most of us very uncomfortable to blame ourselves for a foolish act.

Or you may say, "What a foolish thing I did! I must get in for treatment right away." This is the reasonable approach. Immediate chiropractic care will minimize the effect of the new damage to your body.

Be very careful when you become pain-free. Find out from your chiropractor which activities you can engage in without danger before you begin them. All exercises and body-building programs have their risks. Clear them with him.

When the pain is gone you may talk to yourself a little: "My pain is gone. Everything is better now. I feel fine. Why do I need any more chiropractic adjustments?"

Well, you do. The reason is that in many conditions the pain is gone before the correction is even half completed. The spinal nerve is recovering. The irritation is easing. The interference with the nerve root at the opening between the vertebrae is not great enough to create the pain response. Yet when your chiropractor probes the nerve root, it will still be sore under his fingers. He will find at his fingertips considerable evidence that the structure is still in trouble.

You continue to need chiropractic care until the area of injury has returned to normal, or as near normal as possible. Let your chiropractor tell you when your problem is better. Let him advise you what activities you can enjoy safely and when you need to be treated.

Needless to say, there are patients who terminate treatment when the pain is gone. These are often the people who have an acute problem every year or two, have a few treatments and feel good. They never really get the better of their problem and they do not understand why it gets worse as time goes on. They could have recovered completely at the time of first injury. Now they have developed a chronic, recurring problem that repeatedly hurts. Such a patient's spine often degenerates quietly—as quietly as the rust eating away at his car.

When you are discharged by your chiropractor, your corrective adjustments completed, your pain gone, your areas of structural weakness strengthened, do everything you can to stay well. Remember that the original damage to your spine can be repeated. Spinal correction does not make you immune to future problems, no matter how successful it is. If you put your spine under the same set of conditions that injured it the first time, you may injure it again. Take care of your body!

Ask your chiropractor's advice about exercise and activities to keep your back healthy and strong before you let him discharge you. Your whole body benefits from a healthy spine. Plan to follow his instructions carefully. Exercise regularly. Set apart time for this. Commit yourself to it.

Question your chiropractor about any residual weakness that may have resulted from your injury. Find out if this should be checked regularly. Ask about the possibilities of degenerative changes later in life. If he indicates that there is any permanent change, however small, follow his directions about future checks on it.

Regular examination of the spine a few times a year may save you unnecessary pain when you are older. If you are casual about tooth care, you can always purchase false teeth. You cannot obtain a replacement spine at any price.

I refuse to let my chiropractor discharge me. I want my spine checked every week. Spinal injuries I received in my young years should have crippled me by now. I dove into shallow water and had my hand immediately go numb. I fell from a balcony. I was thrown from a horse, landing on my neck. My X-rays showed permanent damage. Thanks to consistent chiropractic care, I am pain-free; my body is also efficient; my energy level is high. I carry a work load that makes my younger friends feel weary. I can think of no reason for me to terminate the chiropractic care that did this for me.

However, as a chiropractor I discharge patients when they have recovered from an illness and have begun to function at near optimum level. Many people are more interested in maintaining their cars than in maintaining their bodies, and spinal maintenance is always a person's own responsibility. The discharged patient always has the option of returning for periodic adjustments to keep his spine well.

Let me pull a handful of charts from my "Discharged" file and see who got better under chiropractic care. A twenty-year-old man injured his low back and completely recovered. A thirty-five-year-old woman with sinus headaches got complete relief in two weeks of treatment. Two years later she injured her fifth lumbar disc and was treated for five months. A sixty-year-old woman with sciatic pain was treated for a month and recovered.

A thirty-two-year-old man injured his shoulder carrying wood and was treated for a month with full recovery. Three years later he was treated for a low back injury over a two-month period and has had no symptoms for a year.

A four-year-old boy with recurring ear pain and blocking of the tube between the ear and the throat recovered with seven months of treatment, was able to attend school again on a regular basis, and was able to avoid surgery.

A forty-three-year-old man chipping concrete damaged his shoulder after a week of this activity. He recovered with two months of treatment and no time off work.

A thirty-six-year-old woman crushed a vertebra in a tobogganing accident. The fracture healed but pain continued in the area. A year later the patient came to my office in extreme pain and began fifteen months of treatment which restored near normal, pain-free function to the injured spine.

A fifty-year-old whiplash victim was ready for discharge after six weeks of intense treatment.

65

So you're thinking of going to a chiropractor

A young man, sixteen, with a severe headache every few days, had two months' treatment seven years ago. He was discharged with full recovery. I met him a week ago; the pain has not returned.

A thirty-six-year-old man had an occupational injury so severe that he could hardly move. Normal tests were virtually impossible. The previously injured disc was 25 percent of its normal thickness. His son was in for treatment today for a snowmobile accident injury and his wife commented on how well her husband was keeping—no pain, no time off work for the intervening three years.

These statistics may seem repetitive, but they are exciting to a chiropractor. Results built our profession when strong opposing forces were planning and predicting its demise. Today, each time a new patient enters a chiropractor's office anywhere in the world, the uppermost thought in the chiropractor's mind is: "I must find the obstacle to this patient's health. I must discover the key to his recovery."

11

How it all began

THE first chiropractic adjustment to the spine was performed by Daniel David Palmer on September 18, 1895 in the city of Davenport, Iowa. The patient was Harvey Lillard, a hard-working man who injured his spine in a lifting incident, lost his hearing, and was virtually deaf for seventeen years.

After the first adjustment was given, Lillard was able to hear a ticking watch at close range and the rattle of wagons moving down the street outside the building, sounds he had not heard since the time of his spinal injury.

The Reverend Samuel Weed, an early patient of Dr. Palmer and a scholar of Greek and Hebrew, coined the name for the new science. Since adjustment of the spine was administered by hand, he put together the Greek words for "done by hand" and came up with "chiropractic."

Many scientific discoveries happen almost by accident. It was not that way with chiropractic. D. D. Palmer had been searching for years for the underlying cause in human ailments. In his book *The Chiropractor's Adjuster* he wrote: "One question was always uppermost in my mind in my search for the cause of disease. I desired to know why one person was ailing, and his associate, eating at the same table, working in the same shop, at the same bench, was not. Why? What difference was there in the two persons that caused one to have pneumonia, catarrh, typhoid or rheumatism, while his partner, similarly situated, escaped? Why?"

Dr. Palmer himself stressed in his writings that the discovery of chiropractic was not accidental, but rather a product of clear reasoning. In the book quoted above he speaks about the first chiropractic patient: "An examination showed a vertebra racked from its normal position. I reasoned that if that vertebra was replaced the man's hearing would be restored. With this object in view, a half hour's talk persuaded Mr. Lillard to allow me to replace it. I racked it into position using the spinous process as a lever and soon the man could hear as before. There was nothing 'accidental' about this, as

68

it was accomplished with an object in view, and the result expected was obtained."

Dr. Palmer, who had been practicing natural healing methods for a number of years, had a patient soon after with heart trouble. He was not improving with the usual methods he practiced. Dr. Palmer studied the spine in this patient also and records, "I examined the spine and found a displaced vertebra pressing against the nerves which innervate the heart. I adjusted the vertebra and gave immediate relief—nothing 'accidental' or 'crude' about this." He reasoned that if two conditions so different as deafness and heart trouble could be linked to pressure or impingement of nerves, then that might be a common factor in many conditions of the human body.

These simple events that happened before this century began heralded the beginning of chiropractic as a philosophy, an art and a science. The spirit of D. D. Palmer has been found in chiropractors down through the years. Many of the developments in chiropractic have come from thinking men who work with patients every day, analyzing their results, and coming to conclusions that they have been able to pass on for further testing and corroboration in other parts of the world.

Three researchers from the University of Toronto, Merrijoy Kelner, Oswald Hall and Ian Coulter, studied chiropractic in depth. Their report was published in a book, *Chiropractors—Do They Help?* In their report they commented on the times when chiropractic was being discovered by Dr. Palmer.

"At the close of the nineteenth century medical care in the U.S. was far from a flourishing enterprise. Hospitals of the period were poorly equipped to handle illness. Their medical staffs were chosen in a haphazard way. The medical schools of the period, too, were decidedly inadequate. The medical profession itself was torn by dogmatic struggles between the allopaths, the dominant group, and the homeopaths, an insurgent group. The homeopaths vigorously challenged the heavy dosages of drugs in vogue at the time, pointing out that the more modest dosages reduced death rates. It was in this period of poor medical education, meager hospital care, heroic surgery, and heavy doses of drugs that chiropractic emerged as an alternative system of healing." It was a time ripe for the discovery of a safe, conservative approach to health, a way to handle sickness without the risk of massive drug use and inept practitioners.

Daniel D. Palmer was a Canadian, born in 1845 in a log cabin on Lake Scugoge, about thirty miles west of Toronto. At the age of twenty, he emigrated to the United States, established an apiary in New Boston, Illinois, and became one of the largest beekeepers in America. He later moved to Iowa, where he owned a mercantile store in What Cheer. In 1885 he established an office in Davenport and began to give his full time to the study and practice of natural healing methods. He was forty years old.

In 1897 Dr. Palmer was involved in a railroad accident that could have killed him. Suddenly aware of his age and the passing of time, he decided to teach everything he had learned, so that it would not be lost. His first two pupils were physicians named Andrew P. Davis and William A. Seeley, who graduated as Doctors of Chiropractic in 1898.

Like many inventive thinkers, Dr. Palmer had trouble balancing the books, so in 1902 he turned over the administration of the teaching institution, called The Chiropractic School and Cure, to his son Bartlett J. Palmer.

For the next ten years of his life the discoverer of chiropractic traveled, wrote, lectured, and taught in various colleges, some of which he helped found.

B. J. Palmer had the administrative genius that his father lacked. He was thirteen years old when chiropractic was discovered and he became saturated with the study and investigation his father was conducting until, at the age of twenty, he was ready himself to teach. He found his energetic father hard to work with, and in 1906, at the age of twenty-four, bought out his father's share of the college and incorporated the Palmer School of Chiropractic. He was the president from the inception of the Palmer School until his death in 1961.

Chiropractors look on B. J. Palmer as the developer of chiropractic. He received his diploma from the founder in 1902, began teaching at once and produced thirty-seven books of chiropractic insight, reason and thought, meanwhile editing two chiropractic periodicals and building and directing five corporations. One of these was a pioneer broadcasting network, which carried thousands of hours of B. J.'s philosophic and scientific thought, expressed personally by him in his characteristic thought-provoking and charismatic style.

Many in the profession feel that B. J. Palmer's singular dedication to the chiropractic principle that nerve interference leads to disease and the removal of that nerve interference leads to health was a mighty force in keeping chiropractic in its unique position as an alternative healing method to present-day allopathic medicine.

The first chiropractic graduates were dynamic, forward-looking people. Otherwise they would never have had the stamina and endurance to stand up and be counted against the opposition of the establishment of their times.

Solon M. Langworthy established an infirmary in Cedar Rapids, Iowa, but soon converted part of it into a school. In 1903 he named his institution the American School of Chiropractic and Nature Cure. He set up a curriculum for teaching and clinical work for chiropractic education. He established the first chiropractic periodical, *The Backbone,* and wrote a two-volume textbook for chiropractic students in 1906. The first professional organization in chiropractic was also formed by Langworthy. He called it the American Chiropractic Association.

John A. Howard graduated in 1905, served on the faculty of the Palmer School of Chiropractic for a short time, then about 1908, in Davenport, opened the National School, which he later moved to Chicago. He brought university-level professors to teach basic sciences and built patient admissions up to 20,000 a year in the school clinic.

Dr. Willard Carver, a lawyer, was D. D. Palmer's solicitor at the time of the discovery of chiropractic. He advised D. D. in many of the early decisions in the profession. After the founder sold the school to his son, Carver decided to become a chiropractor himself so that he could help guide the developing profession. He had already studied anatomy and physiology at Drake University and took his chiropractic degree at the Charles Ray Parker School of Chiropractic in Oklahoma, graduating in 1906.

How it all began

Dr. Carver did much to stabilize the legislative control of chiropractic and became a prominent educator in the profession. At one time he was president of four colleges simultaneously. He wrote *Carver's Chiropractic Analysis,* a book still valued by chiropractors today. He also developed and taught a unique type of chiropractic adjustive thrust which has stood the test of time.

The list of these noteworthy pioneers of chiropractic is long. Each one made a contribution which is still part of chiropractic as it is practiced to the present, with all the added benefits of decades of experience, insight and subsequent research.

12

Theories that worked

THE early chiropractors used straight-line thinking in their search for an underlying principle of health. The founder of chiropractic reasoned that if a bone in the spine was misplaced before a man went deaf, moving the bone back where it came from should restore the hearing. Then he reasoned that if moving a spinal bone helped a deaf man hear and a heart patient improve, the spine could be the key to improvement in many disease conditions.

He was followed by a number of others who were just as direct in the trip from observation to hypothesis to experiment. They made no attempt to be sophisticated. Getting sick people well was the only matter at hand.

These men lived in an era when the orthodox healers of the day were plagued by confusion in their ranks and ineptness in their methods. There was considerable public concern about this, and the Carnegie Foundation for the Advancement of Teaching commissioned Abraham Flexner to investigate medical education.

Flexner surveyed all 155 medical schools in the United States and Canada and published his results. The *Encyclopaedia Britannica* reports: "His findings, published in 1910 as Bulletin No. 4 of the Carnegie Foundation, resulted in a wholesale closing of the worst of the medical schools and the consolidation and reorganization of others."

Half of the medical schools were closed at the time as a result of the exposure. Flexner recommended that 80 percent should be closed. In his report he made the statement: "For twenty-five years there has been an enormous overproduction of uneducated and ill-trained medical practitioners. This has been in absolute disregard of the public welfare, and without any serious thought of the interests of the public."

People were attracted to medicine by advertising campaigns, moving easily with a few months' preparation from the machine shop to the operating room.

The early chiropractors could easily have gotten a quickie medical diploma and practiced as they pleased. They stood apart, as men of principle, convinced that there was an underlying factor in human disease conditions which they wanted to understand. A number of the early chiropractic students had their osteopathic or medical degrees before they commenced the study of chiropractic.

A recurring concept in the teaching of D. D. Palmer was that disease is an end product of a flaw in body function. In *The Chiropractor's Adjuster,* he made a statement that he repeats often in different ways: "Health is that condition of the body in which all the functions are performed in a normal degree. If they are executed in a too great or too little measure, just in that proportion will there be disease." Later on, he puts it: "Physiologic functions become pathologic when functions are performed in a degree either too great or too little. Therefore we use the term pathologic physiology, meaning abnormal functions."

In that same book Dr. Palmer also claimed to have been the first to pinpoint a number of important principles in medical thought—for example, that life depends upon the condition of nerves, that vertebrae out of alignment impinge upon nerves, and that many disease conditions result from nerve impingement.

The intervening years have been outstanding for scientific achievement. Many of the concepts he presented nearly a century ago are being upheld and advanced by the most respected researchers.

Dr. A. E. Homewood, one of the foremost chiropractic educators of the last forty years and past president of chiropractic colleges in the United States and Canada, writes about D. D. Palmer in one of his books, *The Neurodynamics of the Chiropractic Subluxation:* "Only in recent years have the outstanding scientists of our time been proving the truth of many of D. D. Palmer's principles. The future augurs well for the continued proof of his contentions and the recognition that chiropractic is a method without equal in the correction of the majority of visceral and somatic health problems."

The chiropractor in practice today is just as concerned about the relationships between vertebrae as were the pioneers. There are three basic spinal problems he faces every day.

Fixation involves movement: the normal amount of motion no longer exists between vertebrae. Function has an optimum or normal range, and this loss of motion interferes with the normal balance of health of the components of the intervertebral foramina involved in the area of the fixation.

Dyskinesia is also a disrelationship involving movement, but the movement is greater than normal. At rest, the vertebra appears to be in the normal position; but when the person moves, the vertebra has a bizarre movement pattern, not limited to the normal range.

The *subluxated* vertebra is often an alignment problem, measurable at rest and sometimes painful in action. During the acute phase of a spinal problem, the subluxated vertebra may also be painful at rest.

In all three situations the function of the spine and the contents of the foramina between the involved vertebrae will be affected. Function will change. It will return to normal when the relationships between the vertebrae both at rest and in movement are brought back to normal by chiropractic adjusting.

Nerve receptors are located in the joints between vertebrae, in the ligaments, in the muscles, in the tendons, and in the intervertebral discs. As soon as abnormal

78

movement, tension or placement exists, the message is relayed to the brain and changes take place. Since the messages from one side will differ from those of the other side, the brain will immediately change the function of supporting structures. To restore balance, muscles are tightened and loosened, blood supply is altered and a new awareness exists in both the sensory and the motor areas of the brain relating to the spinal segment. The body works to right itself.

When this situation exists for an extended period of time, the body adjusts itself to the new positioning. Angles in spinal distortion are molded into curves. The head, carried slightly to one side, comes closer to the centered position again, or as close to center as the body can manage.

The irritated nerve becomes fatigued. Junctions between nerves carry impulses across without the usual filtering at the synapse—the non-touching junction between nerves. For a while the neural junctions become overactive but then slow down to a below-normal level of activity. The degenerative processes begin. A chiropractic adjustment is needed.

The theories of D. D. Palmer may have been rudimentary but they were clear and well-defined. His basic concept that disease was a disorder of function was taught in more recent years by the noted Dr. William Boyd. In the preface of his *Text Book of Pathology* he wrote: "Disease in its beginning is abnormal function. Abnormal function is function out of time and phase with environmental need. Disease, whether of the heart, kidney or brain, is disturbed function, not merely disordered structure."

Palmer insisted that disturbances of nerves were

responsible for much disease. It was not a popular idea at the time with the establishment. As the years have passed, there have been fewer and fewer dissenters. In fact the noted Russian neurophysiologist A. D. Speransky was quoted by Dr. J. Janse as saying, "Many pathological processes, the cause of which had been regarded as absolutely foreign to nervous influences, have been found in reality entirely dependent on the latter for their origin."

The teachings of the founder of chiropractic have stood the test of time. His fertile mind produced a mass of written material that is still being investigated and probed. It has not been shot down, as so many of his detractors expected. New discoveries are showing that the path he walked by reason alone was a good one.

Dr. A. E. Homewood comments on this. "The teachings of D. D. Palmer will be found consistent with the facts of our present stage of intellectual insight, and are likely to be found capable of withstanding investigation in the light of new knowledge yet to be discovered —for these are basic truths and principles."

13

A day in a chiropractor's office

YOU may have noticed already that a chiropractor's office is a pleasant place to visit. The whole atmosphere of most offices I have seen seems to breathe the message: "We care about you." The chiropractor and his staff usually work on the principle that people with pain and discomfort should experience as few irritations as possible. Patients under chiropractic care are people, not names or numbers on a chart.

The chiropractor himself finds going to the office a pleasure. A camaraderie exists among his patients, himself and his staff. They share a goal, an anticipation. He enjoys taking his patient from the "nothing can be done" position to one where normal, pain-free action is experienced and internal upsets are corrected. The positive, stimulating challenges he faces every hour keep him alert and tuned in to the latest developments in his profession. Disappointments are kept to a minimum because of the thoroughness of the examining procedures and the exactness of the corrective approaches.

Let me take you through a recent day in my own practice so that you may observe the varied patients who attend a chiropractor. In most of the cases the details will, of necessity, be brief.

My first patient was a lady in her forties who arrived using a cane. The initial examination took place in her home. She had been in bed for eight weeks with an extreme low back problem. The practitioner who had ordered bed rest and drugs did not make house calls, so when she was unable to get out of bed after six weeks, she was in real trouble.

When I first saw this patient she was depressed, frustrated and in extreme pain. It took over a month of treatment to get her pain to a bearable level. Six weeks later we had her on crutches. Now she comes with a cane through all kinds of weather for her spinal correction.

The next patient was a nurse with severe headaches. She was followed by a woman in her seventies who was driven in from another city. Her problem was serious. Degeneration had taken its toll on the lower two verte-

82

brae in the spine and on the discs involved, and she had been in constant pain for several months. When we had examined her and X-rayed her spine, we hesitated to begin until she had committed herself to complete cooperation. We also explained that there was no hope of cure in her case, just freedom from pain with a limited lifestyle if everything went as we expected. She now comes to maintain the correction and relief she obtained during intensive treatment.

A young man who had a history of cervical fracture was next. Movement has been brought virtually to normal in his neck and the dogging consistent pain is gone. Correction is not yet completed.

Two patients drove in together from a country area some distance away. One of them, a beautiful girl in her twenties, had had her life limited by frequent bouts of head pain. The headaches she has now are weeks apart and her posture is slowly improving with correction. Her friend was a former business executive who had decided to run her own business. She had a history of head and neck pain and limitation of movement with pain in her low back. Frequent stomach distress was also a problem. These chronic symptoms are kept in control by chiropractic adjustments. On occasion she has had months with little or no distress.

I saw this first group of patients before breakfast in the office adjoining my home in the country. People who live on farms seldom object to the early hours since it saves them a drive to the city.

My first patient in the city office was a seventy-eight-year-old man who sixty years before had fallen from a haystack to the ground, landing on his head. The telescoping effect of his injuries left him with years of pain. At the time of first examination the patient was in pain all the time. He is in his third month of care. Pain is gone but the correction continues. The young woman who followed had constant pain in the lower back which had been with her for several years. Her father and several members of his family had had surgical repair to their lower backs. To avoid this, she had just begun treatment.

The next three patients had low back problems. One of them was fighting degenerative processes and had trouble in walking, with pain radiating into the hip area. Another had already had surgery but was in great pain. The third had full-blown sciatica. They were followed by a patient with lower cervical distortion in the spine which caused severe arm and shoulder pain from what is known as brachial neuritis.

A young married woman followed; she had been "fighting a cold" and had coughed herself into pain in her back and around her ribs. As we corrected the spinal problem the cold began to improve. This always amazes people, but chiropractors see it happen too often to be surprised. She was followed by an interesting young man who had been thrown from a motorcycle fifteen feet into the air, landed on top of a car and then dropped onto the road. We were just beginning correction and he was in pain.

The next five patients were women with nerve root irritation in the lower neck, middle lumbar, mid-thoracic, lumbosacral and upper thoracic areas of the spine respectively. One of the ladies had had serious infection of the mandible and was also treated for a faulty function of the temporomandibular joint, which hinges the lower jaw. The infection was history when

84

she consulted me, but her jaw had frequently locked until she began having chiropractic manipulative correction. The frightful locking has not taken place since correction began.

The middle-aged man who followed her has an advanced low back problem which he refuses to believe is serious. He will disappear from the patient roster as soon as the pain is gone, I am sure, and will go through the whole process again in a few months. It's a hard way to go, but some choose that course.

A woman in her thirties was next. She had been told she had osteoarthritis and did in fact have severe pain in several joints. No bony change showed on X-ray examination, but she had an oblique pelvic tilt, her cervical spine had lost its normal curve and there were subluxated vertebrae in all three sections of her spine. The lumbar distortion also related to the numbness she had in two toes of her right foot.

Next was a young man with acute low back pain, then a pensioner with degeneration of his lowest spinal disc, then a woman who had been injured at work. Then came a most delightful lady in her seventies with severe heart trouble, who needed help with her arthritis and the circulation in her legs. She smiled widely as she mentioned that sharp leg pains in the night had disappeared. A woman with chronic foot pain followed.

A woman with extreme headaches that nothing could change came next, saying that she had not had a headache since her last visit. The next patient also had headaches, but these were only on one side of the head. They had been paining more or less for ten years. The effect on the patient was seen mostly in her eyes. She looked as if she was peering through binoculars. As her

85

headaches eased, her thoracic spine became painful. Her real problem will not be cleared until a pelvic distortion is corrected, which is probably the result of a fall during childhood or her teen years. This will take time but she can anticipate freedom from her head pain in the future.

The next patient was an elderly lady whose right hip and leg pain was gone, but who could not understand that her spinal problem was not yet reduced to a safe level of correction. We had a little talk, but I am not sure how much good it did. She was followed immediately by a man who had had surgical repair to an injured hip which makes him walk slightly lopsided. He is semi-retired and remains pain-free by having his off-balance lower back adjusted periodically. The next patient, has had back injury in the past. He came in for a routine check on his spine. Another patient with arm and neck pain was waiting.

A former patient who had just injured her lumbar spine arrived in great pain and feeling nausea and stomach distress. When the examination was completed, I first relieved the abdominal symptoms by adusting the fifth thoracic vertebra. Then I lifted the pressure from the damaged disc and sent the patient home to apply ice to the area; ice minimizes the swelling and helps limit the possibility of permanent damage.

A very buoyant woman of about forty was prepared and waiting for treatment. She complained of "prickly feet," which was her way of saying that pins-and-needles sensations in her feet and legs were a great concern to her. Her first examination showed spinal nerve involvement in the lower lumbar spine. Her history included an auto accident nine years before and a fall down the stairs three years before, and she had lifted a heavy mattress by herself on the day the symptoms appeared. It took a month of steady correction before the improvement began.

A lady with arthritic knees who now walks without pain came next, then a young man with a posture problem. Two whiplash victims from the same accident followed; mother and son had been injured, but no one had taken their injuries seriously. After a cursory medical examination they had been told that nothing was wrong. Four months later, in extreme pain that had kept them awake nights, they came to me for treatment. The son will completely recover. The mother has permanent damage. When I finally persuaded her to retain a lawyer, she began to get all kinds of help, specialists became involved, alternate treatment methods were suggested, injections were advised. She continues to improve with chiropractic adjustments.

Two men came in with stress symptoms from overwork and from attempting to keep up with a very heavy schedule. After examination, one was relieved with treatment; the other had systemic lupus erythematosis, for which he had sought medical care. He was advised after treatment to ease his pace and satisfy the nutritional needs associated with his condition. A patient with constant diarrhea and blood in the stool was treated next. Her condition had gone on for weeks, and it had not responded to the drugs prescribed for it. The history indicated that the patient had just returned from a trip abroad. I advised her on what to eat and adjusted her spine. Within two days she was greatly improved. Her allopathic specialist was pleased with the changes and told her to follow my nutritional instructions for a long period. Teamwork was valuable in her case.

87

A business executive then came with acute low back pain, followed by a nurse with a recurring low back problem from too much lifting and pain in the rib cage—intercostal neuralgia.

Two people with disc injuries followed, one of whom had had low back surgery but had experienced excruciating low back pain which radiated down his leg to the foot when he first visited this office. He is now without pain but continues needing correction.

A patient with some degenerative changes in her spine that are being controlled came next, then a woman who struggles with her tension but finds relief with chiropractic adjustments. A man then arrived from another city who first came to this office with chest pain and extreme fatigue. He maintains the health he now enjoys by a weekly spinal check, and doesn't mind the travel it calls for. We then treated a patient with pain between the shoulders, a patient with low back injury, and a patient who had had a penetrating wound in the spine, who keeps energetic and almost pain-free with chiropractic care. Two low back injuries followed.

A couple arrived together who had been in a head-on automobile accident. The husband is in constant head pain with what has been diagnosed as an aneurysm, or enlargement of a blood vessel in the brain. I have not been able to help his head pain, but the middle and lower spine, painful from severe injuries through the years, we have been able to help. His wife had a kyphotic development in the upper thoracic spine after her accident. This is steadily improving.

A patient with a low back distortion in the final stages of correction followed, then a patient with marked degeneration involving the two lowest lumbar discs.

A day in a chiropractor's office

The next patient had fallen through a trapdoor and down a flight of stairs several months ago. She had many consultations and months of physiotherapy before coming for examination and chiropractic adjustments to her neck and spine. As we began, she was in extreme pain, but she is now beginning to recover.

Three members of one family were together: father and mother for spinal correction and their son for an acute hockey injury to his pelvis and lower back. A whiplash victim followed them.

A thirty-nine-year-old woman who looked ten years younger came in with the complaint that she had had low back pain for years, had had many tests and examinations, had been hospitalized recently for X-rays and injections and had tried acupuncture, all without success. Today was her tenth visit and she had been two days without pain. Another patient of the same age followed who had been in an auto accident a year before and had had constant pain in her right arm, which frequently went numb. She could tilt her head only fifteen degrees instead of forty degrees either way. She has been under treatment six months and is running a successful hairdressing business. A patient with acute lumbar pain followed.

My next patient was an actor of considerable repute with frequent stomach disorders and trigeminal neuralgia or, as it is commonly known, tic douloureux. He also had had right shoulder and neck pain. After ten days of treatment he was about sixty percent improved and producing a play that is expected to be a sellout.

A patient with ligamentous damage and a consequently recurring low back problem was waiting; then a young lady who had been through extreme back pain appeared for her biweekly adjustment. A woman with neck and arm pain followed, who was recovering very quickly because her nutrition had been maintained at a good level for years; the damaged tissues had everything they needed to heal.

A patient with cancer was next. I am not treating her for cancer. Tissue damage was so great in this patient that a simple act like reaching for a telephone would leave her in extreme pain. Gentle manipulation of the spinal segments helped her through another day. Though only fifty-one, she does not object to dying but she resents the pain that plagues her with any unthinking movement.

An accountant was next who had knee pains and pins-and-needles sensation in her right hip area which had made it very difficult for her to sit down to do her work. She had visited another practitioner without success, but had the courage to try again. Her condition is slowly changing and she now has no difficulty sitting all day at her desk.

A patient with arthritic changes in his spine and chronic back pain was next. He is a candidate for bypass surgery and knows that some of his heart arteries are functioning poorly, but he resists the surgery and the stress is making his pain worse.

I moved from him to a man in his late twenties who has a problem with high blood pressure. No medication seemed to lower it, so his medical doctor gave him a prescription to slow his heartbeat from the normal 72 beats per minute to about 45 beats per minute. He had been on this for some time and became concerned that this would be his life pattern. I explained to him some of the natural approaches to blood pressure control and began to give him spinal adjustments. We charted his blood pressure weekly. I assured him that the practitioner who gave the prescription would most certainly reduce the dosage or eliminate it if that seemed indicated. As I checked his blood pressure a few weeks later, I noticed that his pulse and his blood pressure were normal. When I commented on this, the patient advised me that he had self-terminated the use of the drug, which of course is his prerogative. The situation has continued for a month now, blood pressure normal, pulse normal; not a bad way to go through life, even if it does take a chiropractic adjustment a week for a few months. His wife commenced treatment for a spinal problem and was my next patient.

I then treated a patient with an unusual rotation of some of the lower thoracic vertebrae. She had been working extremely hard and had sustained some blows to her back. She was already improving after only a few adjustments. She was followed by an accident victim in his second year of corrective manipulation.

A former player on the Calgary Stampeders football team was waiting for treatment. Athletes are hard on themselves and each other and he was no exception. I adjusted old injuries to his neck and low back.

A housewife with stress symptoms and pain between the shoulders and a young lady in her twenties with knee problems rounded out the day in the office.

I visited only three patients in their homes on the day I have chosen to describe. The first I saw on the way to the city office. He is a gentleman in his eighties with weakness in one of the muscles attached to the shoulder blade and a lower thoracic kyphosis. My visit to his home is always a pleasure, and I consider him a dear friend.

During the lunch hour I saw a lady who has been more or less crippled since 1938—over forty years. With both hips rigid, she has very limited mobility with crutches. Her life has contained years of pain. As the pain diminished under chiropractic adjustments, she began to hope she might take some steps again—hope, at eighty years old. I assured her that it was enough of a wonder that the pain was easing without expecting a miracle. I joked with her that I did not like too many miracles, because everyone lined up for repeats. It was a happy visit.

The other lunch-hour patient was a woman who fights arthritis in the spine, shoulders and hands. Though she is just approaching middle age, she has endured pain for years. Her days are pleasant now, and there are no signs that the condition has progressed since we began treatment about a year ago.

A heavy case load such as I carry is not unusual for a chiropractor. When the original information has been carefully gathered, and the treatment plan prepared, the actual correction of a troubled spinal area is accomplished by a series of gentle adjustments. Examinations are time-consuming, but the actual spinal adjustment on a visit to your chiropractor may take only a few moments.

When the last patient left the office, I sat down to write one of the earlier chapters of this book. There is not much time for writing in a chiropractor's day, but I wanted to communicate some of the basics that make chiropractic work.

It seems important, too, to say that chiropractic practice is demanding, exacting and exhausting, but it is one of the greatest ways to spend your life that I can think of.

My son said to me recently, "Dad, you enjoy practice so much that I think you should pay the patients who come to you instead of having them pay."

Maybe he's right!

14

Your fascinating nervous system

A NEW human life is conceived when the male sperm penetrates the resistance of the cell wall of the female ovum. Immediately the newly formed cell begins to grow. One cell becomes two. Two cells become four. Four cells become eight. The new entity goes on this way for twenty-one days, growing just as a cancer cell grows, with no control from the brain of either parent, the growth fostered by the abundant presence of estrogen.

On the twenty-first day the cells that will ultimately become the pancreas give the tiniest imaginable spurt of trypsin. This counters the effect of the estrogen and stops its action instantly. From that time on, the growth is under the control of the primitive streak, an unusual name given to the cells that will form the brain and nervous system in the growing body.

The human nervous system contains more than ten billion nerve cells. These form an intricate, detailed, widespread network of communicating fibers which keep the brain in touch with all the tissue cells of the body. A thread of nerve reaches to the site of every cell except those floating freely in the body fluids.

The basic unit of the nervous system is the neuron or nerve cell, which is usually pictured as a small body with a tail which may be as much as a yard in length. On the opposite side of the nerve cell body a group of shorter projections called dendrites are located.

Normally, a nerve impulse enters the nerve cell through the dendrites, passes through the cell nucleus and moves on down the axon to the next relay center. This may be a synapse, or junction point where the nerve impulse enters another nerve cell. It may also enter a muscle, gland or other tissue cell and stimulate that cell to do what it does. A muscle cell will be stimulated to contract. A gland cell will be stimulated to secrete.

Nerve energy moves along the nerve fiber in a way that compares with the way electricity moves along a wire. The nerve impulse has an electrical voltage which is used to transmit the nerve impulse. The energy in the

96

nerve impulse is never transmitted to other structures such as the stomach, heart, muscles or glands. The impulse is simply used to trigger the action the ultimate action cell performs.

The nerve impulse can be compared to the match that sets off a dynamite explosion. The match is the trigger that makes it happen, but it does not contribute to the force of the explosion.

When a muscle receives an impulse from its associated nerves, the force of the contraction depends on the number of cells receiving the impulse, the number of impulses received per second, and the ability of the muscle cells to contract.

The moment your finger touches a hot burner on your stove, a microscopic sense organ in the deep skin is stimulated. This is attached to a nerve cell that travels toward the spinal cord and makes a relay connection with the brain where other contacts are made. When the impulse is received in the sensory area of the brain, you become aware of the burning sensation. Another action, initiated in the spinal cord through two different nerve cells, relays the message to appropriate muscles so that the finger is withdrawn from the burner by the time the brain knows that the burner is hot.

If you remove the brain from the skull, it looks like a giant walnut. It is the surface area with all its rough ins and outs that makes possible the superior intelligence of animals and humans. The weight of the human brain also gives man an edge. A man with a large head is not necessarily more intelligent than a smaller person; it is the surface area of the brain and how it is being used that counts.

The central nervous system includes the brain and

spinal cord. It is well protected by the skull and spinal vertebrae. The unique structure of the spinal bones allows for maximum movement. With proper care, the full movement can be maintained right into advanced age. With abuse, movement becomes limited and often painful as the normal movement between spinal segments is lost. Often several vertebrae will become fixed and move like one piece, to the detriment of the joints at the end of the area of fixation.

The bony protective covering of the brain and spinal cord is effective and valuable, but if it is ever penetrated or broken, any damage to nerve tissue will be permanent.

When a person is paralyzed from an accident, part of the paralysis will be not from nerve tissue damage but from inflammation of the area, from swelling and from alteration of the normal blood supply. The function of damaged tissues can sometimes be taken over by another part of the central nervous system. The only permanent damage that cannot improve is nerve cell destruction.

Certain parts of the brain have clearly defined functions. Just above the ear there is a strip that goes to the top of the head on each side which, when active, makes the muscles of the body accomplish useful work. It is called the motor strip. Behind this and more or less parallel to it is the sensory strip which receives sensations from all parts of the body.

The back of the brain contains the visual area where sensations from the eye are received and evaluated. Halfway forward on each side of the brain is an area where we receive and interpret impulses from the ear.

Most of the motor fibers from the right side of

98

the brain cross over to the left side and produce activity on the left side of the body, and vice versa. These nerve fibers pass down the spinal cord to the level of action. They link with other nerve cells and the lower motor neurons pass out of the cord in the spinal nerve which passes through two matched notches composing the intervertebral opening chiropractors measure and manipulate. This opening on each side at each level of the spine is called the intervertebral foramen. Irritation, impingement and interference with the spinal nerve at this point can cause many problems.

The body basically functions in slices. The spinal nerve at each level looks after the slice at that level. From the spinal nerve two branches form, a sensory branch taking impulses into the rear portion of the cord, and a motor branch taking impulses out of the front portion of the cord. In the cord itself, tracts of fibers carrying similar impulses are grouped together in a most orderly fashion.

The nervous system enables the body to use several functions together to adapt to its environment. Think of posture for a moment. The soles of the feet send information through the sensory nerves to the brain. The visual information from the eyes is added to this by the brain. In the inner ear, the vestibular apparatus, a system of tubes with liquid in them, is influenced by movements of the head, and this information is correlated with the rest. A constant flow of information is received from joints and muscles. All this information passes through the thalamus, the switchboard for signals going to and from the brain. It is relayed to the computer-like cerebellum which controls the coordination of our movements and advises the motor center of the cerebrum where we need a little more or less muscle tone to maintain our normal stance.

There are areas of the brain which can be removed with little or no effect on normal life activities. When a person has a stroke, he has a lack of blood supply, or an application of pressure to a part of the brain or to the pathways leading to or from the brain.

Recovery from a stroke sometimes seems to border on the miraculous. There is a reason for this. While some of the damaged brain cells are dead within as little as four minutes if their oxygen supply is cut off, this area of destruction may be quite small. The surrounding area may be affected so that it refuses to function, or so that it functions poorly but is not permanently damaged. The cells are not dead. Most patients who suffer from a stroke, medically called a cerebrovascular accident or CVA, should be treated optimistically. The quicker the signs of recovery, the better the final outcome will likely be. Only a minority die quickly, usually due to continuing hemorrhage that cannot be stopped and progressively destroys brain tissue by pressure.

The junction between two nerve cells is called the synapse. It links the axon of one nerve with the dendrites of another. The synapse contains a chemical transmitter substance; acetylcholine is a common one. The transmitter substance allows the nerve impulse to jump the gap between the two nerve cells which do not touch. The axons, sometimes three feet in length, are insulated by a sheath from other axons in the same nerve trunk.

A nerve impulse speeds down an axon. When it arrives at the end, the chemical transmitter stored there is released in a quick blast between the two cells. The

100

impulse jumps the gap and travels through the next nerve cell. Immediately the transmitter substance is replaced at the end of the axon so that the next impulse, coming a split second later, can get across. It all happens with such speed that it would be impossible to accomplish the feat mechanically.

Nerve cells contain only the tiniest amount of chemical transmitter at the end of their axons, just enough for a few minutes of normal life activity. The body is continuously forming this transmitter substance at every synapse in the body. In his book *Functions of the Human Body,* physiologist Arthur C. Guyton, M.D. speaks of some axons firing across the synapse two to three hundred times in a second.

Another amazing thing about the synapse is that it allows the impulse to cross only in one direction. After an impulse flashes from one nerve cell to another, the synapse is unable to conduct anything across for one two-thousandth of a second. The impulse that crossed the synapse cannot come back.

Under repeated stimulation a synapse will begin to get tired and lose its effectiveness. The supply of chemical transmitter becomes exhausted and the synapse rests. This is particularly important during an epileptic seizure. Many synapses are bombarded with great excitability and stimulation. Gradually the seizure subsides; the synapses have become fatigued.

Frequent excitation of synapses over a period of days with the same kind of stimulation causes a change in the shape and size of the terminals over which the repeated impulses have passed; the number of terminals will also increase. This is thought to be part of the basis of memory. Parallel stimuli moving across the same

101

synapses for a period of time convince the body that these nerve pathways are important. The innate intelligence of the body makes a structural change in the synapses so that these may be stimulated much more easily than before.

Once the memory circuit has been established, it appears to continue without change even after the stimulation no longer passes over that route. Years later it is possible to bring the memory back and reactivate the pathway by stimulating the part of the cerebral cortex where the information had been stored. This is why you may go for years without riding a bicycle and then easily do it again without learning a second time.

As we get older, the number of synapse terminals between nerve cells in the cerebral cortex greatly increases. We keep on, throughout our lifetime, building new pathways of memory. The seventy-year-old person may have up to fifteen trillion pieces of information stored in his memory, according to an estimate made by a neurophysiologist at the University of Michigan. On the other hand, if we totally stop using some pathways in the brain, that part of the brain tends to get thinner. This has been noted particularly in animals that have lost their sight; the visual portion of the brain thinned markedly because it was not being used at all.

Buried in the skin throughout the surface of the body are microscopic nerve receptors. Each receptor is unique and can receive only one kind of sensation. Pain receptors number three to four million. Touch receptors number about half a million, and pressure is linked with these as prolonged touch. Two hundred thousand temperature sensor organs are present, recording heat or cold. A single nerve cell picks up the sensation in each

102

receptor and whisks the impulse to the spinal cord; it is then relayed to the brain.

Motor impulses returning from the brain are carried to the level of the cord involved and are then relayed to the muscle or other tissue cell. When the nerve contacts a muscle fiber, there is an end plate, which is a fairly complicated structure, reaching into the muscle but separate from it.

A nerve impulse reaches the junction between nerve and muscle; the nerve fiber releases a chemical transmitter; the muscle contracts. Another substance immediately destroys the chemical transmitter. It has only two thousandths of a second to do its work. In myesthenia gravis the nerve impulse gets right to the end of the nerve fiber but cannot get into the muscle cell.

The nervous system is both marvelous and complicated. We have only scratched the surface here; there is another side of it that is wholly automatic, called the autonomic nervous system. Always keep in mind that you are functioning right now only as well as your nervous system is functioning.

How will you feel the next time a well-meaning practitioner with only drugs to give you says, "It is just your nerves that are causing your trouble. I'll give you a tranquilizer to calm them down. You will feel better."

Is that the kind of treatment you want? It is true that nerves are involved in almost every human illness. You may even feel better for a while. If tranquilizers treat only symptoms, where will you go when you stop the drug and return to your undrugged state? Some people stay on tranquilizers for years. Would you do that?

Feeling better is not the only goal of treatment.

103

To soothe is not always to cure. When the intricacies of the nervous system are involved, it is important to you that the cause of your problem be found and corrected, if that is at all possible.

In his book *A Look at Chiropractic Spinal Correction* Dr. I. N. Toftness states, "The discovery that interference in the operation of the human nervous system could be precipitated by minor luxations in the human skeletal framework was dramatic, for the reason that the nervous system controls the physical body. . . . The nervous system can keep a body well or make it sick, depending on the way it is treated by its owner. . . . It is the nervous system that plays the major role in physiological function."

Every time a chiropractor adjusts a spine, he influences the nervous structures in and around that spine. It is the most direct approach that can be used to reduce nerve interference at the openings through which spinal nerves leave the spinal column.

15

Your chiropractor's nutritional concerns

FOOD is important to you. It is the building material by which your body is maintained. The food you ate yesterday is present today as body cells, blood, lymph fluid, hormones and enzymes. It gave you the energy to keep active in the hours since it was eaten. Every time a muscle moves, a gland secretes or a nerve discharges an impulse, energy from food is used up.

Different body cells require different nutrition. Their function is specialized and so is their diet. The thyroid gland needs iodine to function; nerve tissue is hungry for the B vitamins; bones need a sustained supply of minerals; your skin needs vitamin A; the heart constantly requires potassium.

All these must be supplied by your intake of food. If your personal diet does not include the nutrients requested by the body cells, in the quantities they are using, then some of the cells will suffer from malnutrition and will weaken. They will become sick cells, and their resistance to invaders will be lessened. And yet you may be unaware of any lack of nourishment—you may even be overweight, eating the wrong foods because you learned to eat that way or were drawn into it by attractive and seductive advertising.

Your chiropractor adjusts your spine to balance the function of body systems and restore health. He is well equipped to do this. If you ask him, he will tell you that results are consistently better in bodies that have received good nutrition. Healthy cells, when injured, recover more quickly than cells that are missing needed nutrients. The empty-calorie foods often give you brief energy boosts while your cells get weaker.

Obtaining good nutrition is not complicated. You need to understand a few principles and to be consistent in applying them. There is no need to suffer from poor nutrition.

Start with the basics. Food consists of three basic substances: carbohydrates, fats and protein.

Carbohydrates are all around us. They are the easiest foods to obtain. Simple carbohydrates like sugar and bleached white flour are not helpful to us; refining hurts them and then they hurt us. A diet heavy in sugar overworks the pancreas and may result in exhausting it. If you avoid simple carbohydrates and eliminate white sugar and bleached flour from your diet, you will take a giant step toward good nutrition.

Complex carbohydrates are excellent foods. They includes vegetables, whole grains and fruits. These digest more slowly than simple carbohydrates and keep a level supply of energy available to the body.

Fats are also easy to find. You may eat a steak for its protein content without thinking that at least thirty percent of it is fat. We have the habit of spreading fat on our bread in the form of butter or margarine. Animal fats are mostly saturated fats. These are the hardest fats for the body to handle.

Whenever we need fat to cook with, we would do well to use unsaturated oil from vegetable sources, such as safflower oil, peanut oil, soybean oil and corn oil. These will provide the fat our body needs for normal functioning and also contain essential fatty acids which are a part of every body cell.

The essential fatty acids are thought to be used in the body to make a substance called lecithin which is required to control cholesterol deposits on the blood vessels and to keep cholesterol molecules from forming harmful clumps in the circulating blood.

Lecithin is a phospholipid found in the soybean which is used in the digestion of fats in the body. It is widely found in nature, but since it is often immediately under the skin of fruits and vegetables, much of it is thrown away when we refine and cook our food. Lecithin makes up twenty to thirty percent of the brain substance in a normal adult, over forty percent in geniuses and less than twenty percent in retarded peoples.

Protein is found in meat, fish, fowl and eggs, and also in milk, yeast, beans and nuts. Protein is essential for growth and tissue repair. All of the body tissues are protein—glands, skin, muscle, eyes, blood, nails, even hair.

Protein is made up of substances called amino acids, of which there are at least twenty-two. Eight of these cannot be manufactured in the body, and are called essential amino acids because they must be taken in in food. In fact, they must all be taken together in a single meal to make the protein required for repairs. Otherwise the protein intake may be burned off as so many calories for energy. This is a terrible waste of a vital resource.

If I had to choose only one supplement to my diet, my first choice would be a soybean protein with added calcium sodium caseinate to bring the methionine up to the level of the other seven essential amino acids. A single ounce in a glass of milk is quite palatable. This protein, taken first thing in the morning, raises my blood sugar from the sleep level to the level for normal activity and keeps it there for hours. Protein is needed in the morning for normal hormone development and function and normal enzyme activity to get under way. Enzymes and hormones are protein substances and are absolutely vital to the body's metabolic activities. When all the essential amino acids are present at once, as many as twelve thousand natural antibodies are formed and kept in action. These substances give us powerful resistance to disease.

The morning lag that follows a breakfast of simple

108

carbohydrates usually hits around eleven o'clock. Protein in the morning virtually eliminates this. The blood sugar level remains steady. Factories put in coffee breaks to overcome the rash of accidents caused by the mid-morning energy drop. Morning protein is a better way.

The question is, can we survive with optimum health just by making sure that our diets are adequate in the supply of carbohydrates, fats and proteins?

Many researchers and authorities say, "No!"

Robert J. Benowicz, in his national bestseller *Vitamins and You,* says: "Although contemporary foods retain measurable and predictable amounts of protein, carbohydrate and fat, chemical and physical manipulation plays havoc with their vitamin and mineral stores."

Nathan Pritikin writes in his book *The Pritikin Program for Diet and Exercise,* "The convenience food diet most Americans live by . . . is faddish and reckless. Our systems are plainly uncomfortable with the chemical hocus-pocus that parades as, or invades, our food supply. In one way or another, some 3500 new chemicals have found their way into our food—and common sense tells us that our bodies simply aren't ready for them."

In *Earl Mindell's Vitamin Bible* we are told emphatically, "Most of the food we eat has been processed and depleted in nutrients."

Doctors R. G. Mazlen and L. E. Bradshaw wrote in their book *Nutrition and Your Health,* "One of the most prevalent modern myths is that three so-called 'balanced meals' invariably provide adequate overall nutritional values for anyone—regardless of age, sex, occupation, state of health or energy output. This over-simplified claim lulls the unknowing or confused con-

109

sumer into a false sense of security. Nutritional survey data document that even affluent Americans can become undernourished in the dogmatic pursuit of the 'three square meals' theory."

These authorities agree that the modern North American diet needs help. Our attempts to make food taste better and to keep it from spoiling have damaged our source of nutrition. We must recapture some of the vitamins and minerals that have been lost in the shuffle.

Since these vital factors are food substances, they can be mixed and taken together, just as we do with other foods. A number of reliable suppliers have prepared multivitamin and mineral combinations from all natural sources. If these are added to meals, you can restore your nutrition to the normal level that your body should enjoy for good health. These vitamins and minerals supplement the nutritionally deficient food. That is why the name "food supplements" is often used to describe them.

My personal supplementation program includes vitamin A because it is valuable for skin, eyes and the membranes of the whole intestinal tract. It is derived from fish liver oil, but in combination with other substances the taste is not evident.

The B vitamins I consider specially important because as a group they equip me for the strenuous life I like to lead. They are great stress aids. Take a quick look at them.

B1 is called thiamine. It assists in the conversion of food into energy, aids in rebuilding liver cells, is vital to brain cells and memory and to nerve cells in general.

B2 is named riboflavin and helps form various hormones in the body, notably growth hormones, adrenal hormones including ACTH, metabolic hormones and insulin.

B3 is niacin, which increases surface capillary blood flow, acts as a coenzyme for food metabolism, is important to the function of the central nervous system, has a regulating effect on hormone production and assists in the formation of bile salts in the body.

B5 is also known as pantothenic acid and functions as a coenzyme for metabolism in the cells of the body, aids in the production of chemical transmitters for nerve impulses, helps the adrenal glands to perform well and controls histamine reactions.

B6 or pyridoxine is required to form proteins from amino acids and to form fats from fatty acids, builds immunity to disease, controls formation of niacin, red blood cells and some hormones. It aids in the chemical balance of body fluids and influences water excretion from the body.

B12 or cobalamin became well known in the control of pernicious anemia. It works with folic acid to regulate red blood cells and the formation of genetic materials. It is a coenzyme in the formation of RNA and DNA for the rebuilding of body cells and formation of new cells.

Folic acid is involved in the formation and health of the nervous system. It maintains the sex organs, white blood cells and growth patterns and helps synthesize the RNA and DNA molecules.

Biotin is also included in the B complex. It aids the metabolism of unsaturated fatty acids, builds body tissue, and maintains sweat glands, nerve tissue, bone marrow, male sex glands, blood cells, skin and hair.

Choline is another B factor which assists memory

storage, moves substances across cell membranes, and makes acetylcholine for movement of the nerve impulse across the synapse. In a test mentioned by Adelle Davis in her book *Let's Get Well,* 158 patients with high blood pressure showed improvement while taking choline and also showed notable strengthening of the capillary walls while the supplement was being taken.

The B vitamins are good for stress because they tune up the adrenals and liver and assist in the metabolism of all cells. They also aid red blood cell formation and help regulate the heartbeat. They are very important in the transmission of the nerve impulse from one neuron to another.

Good sources of the B vitamins are liver, organ meats, yeast, wholegrain cereals, wheat germ, soybeans, peanuts and fresh fish, but it is often necessary to supplement your diet with B complex.

Each morning I also take 1000 milligrams of vitamin C in a timed-release tablet. This means that throughout the day I have a sustained inner protection from this valuable food. This vitamin C is called "natural" and includes some of the substances normally associated with vitamin C when it is found in nature. It comes from vegetable sources, rather than being synthesized in a lab as man attempts to mimic nature.

Vitamin C is an important item in the human diet because it is known to help the body fight infections. When a germ attacks a body cell, a substance is released to break down the cement that holds the cells together. This opens up a path for the spread of the invader.

The body immediately begins its program of repair. As the barriers to infection are built up again, vitamin C supplies some of the needed materials from which the cell cement is made. The infection may be limited or stopped if there is enough vitamin C in the tissues.

Storage of vitamin C in the body is limited. What is needed today must be in today's diet. If an invader strikes when the vitamin C level in your body is low, you may become needlessly susceptible to the infection. It has been found that using timed-release vitamin C may increase the quantity in body tissues by as much as four times.

Chiropractors have known for many years that vitamin C fights infections. It was taught in my undergraduate class in 1953, based on extensive research already done.

The value of vitamin C has been established in extremely well-controlled studies by researchers using standard scientific methods in their work. Many double-blind studies have been done. Yet Dr. Linus Pauling, Nobel prize winner and a medical researcher of international repute, wrote in the preface to the revised edition of his book *Vitamin C, the Common Cold, and the Flu* that in 1974 ". . . most physicians and authorities in the field of nutrition continued to describe vitamin C as having no value in controlling the common cold, or any other disease, except its specific deficiency disease, scurvy."

In his introduction to the same book, Dr. Pauling makes a claim based on his study of the available results of vitamin C research: "It is my opinion now, after an additional six years of study in this field, that for most people the improvement in health associated with the ingestion of the optimum amount of ascorbic acid is not just such as to lead to an increase in life expectancy by only four to six years; instead, my present estimate is

113

that the increase probably lies in the range twelve to eighteen years." If vitamin C has the potential to add to our years of life, it is well worth noticing.

My daily food supplement includes minerals. Since minerals are a little harder than other substances for the body to assimilate, I use chelated minerals. This simply means that amino acids are already attached to the mineral ions and together they form a molecule which is easily absorbed through the intestine into the bloodstream.

This chelation of minerals should take place in the intestine, but experience has shown that many minerals pass through the mouth that never pass into the bloodstream. *Earl Mindell's Vitamin Bible* claims that "only about 8 percent of your total iron intake is absorbed and actually enters your bloodstream." One wag made the comment that many mineral tablets enter the mouth, navigate the digestive tract and leave the body with the trademark still visible on the tablet.

Chelated minerals are prepared in advance to be absorbed into the blood so that the body can use them. This is worth knowing since the body can put some vitamins together for itself, but all its minerals must come from the outside. Notice the importance of a few of them.

Calcium is the most abundant body mineral. It forms the bones and teeth, but also helps regulate the heartbeat, facilitates the transmission of nerve impulses, aids the clotting of blood as required and keeps muscles from becoming irritable and cramping.

Magnesium is an antistress mineral which aids in nerve and muscle function, including the heart action, and helps to convert blood sugar to energy.

Phosphorus is found in every body cell and is a

vital factor in the proteins of the cell nucleus. It helps to form strong teeth and bones, is used in fat and carbohydrate metabolism and is found in the insulating sheaths of nerve fibers.

Potassium works with sodium to move nutrients across cell membranes and to regulate body fluids. It helps keep body fluids alkaline, stimulates the kidneys, helps store sugars as glycogen and keeps the adrenals healthy.

Iron enables the red blood cells to carry oxygen and is in each cell to enable it to use oxygen and to receive it from the body fluids. It also assists in B vitamin metabolism and in synthesis of proteins for tissue repair.

Chromium is important for keeping tissues elastic and youthful. It has been found to reverse atherosclerosis and assists the metabolism of sugar. In the male it is concentrated in the prostate and sexual channels.

Manganese aids normal bone structure, promotes proper use of glucose and aids cholesterol and lipid synthesis. It activates enzymes, prevents sterility and helps the pancreas in both its development and its function.

Zinc maintains the acid–alkaline balance, makes the brain function efficiently, stimulates healing and is a component of insulin. It is essential for B complex absorption, for nucleic acid synthesis, for white blood cell production, for normal prostate function and for reproduction.

The minerals are so vital to body functions that if you are at all health-conscious you will want to consider them in your plans for good health in the future. Do not assume that you have enough of each. Make sure of it!

115

16

Questions patients ask their chiropractors

THE very nature of a chiropractic practice makes it impossible to answer every question a patient might want to ask. This is regrettable because it is a pleasure for a chiropractor to talk about his profession. I have had patients write their queries down so that they would remember what to ask. These people got their questions answered. Many others have found that the adjustment was over and

So you're thinking of going to a chiropractor

I had moved on before they thought of what they wanted to ask, and by the next visit they had forgotten it. I do have the habit, though, of talking most of the time while I work, so a patient's questions are often answered before they are asked. It is my pleasure now to share with you some of the questions frequently heard by a chiropractor.

Can you cure my problem?

Every chiropractor in the world would like to cure every patient. There is tremendous satisfaction in a completed job. This is often possible, even in acute cases. Many of the cases that come to a chiropractor have been on the way to trouble for a long time. The final slip or twist that started the sustained pain just brought the weakness to the patient's attention.

It is no advantage to a patient to push a developing problem back under the level of pain because it will return. The recurrences often get worse each time. Sometimes changes in the spine have gone too far to be completely reversed, but it is of great benefit to the patient to bring it as close to normal as possible.

What is the clicking sound I sometimes hear when my spine is adjusted?

When a vertebra is adjusted with a chiropractic thrust, it makes a slight gliding movement along the joint surfaces, which part slightly. There are no empty spaces in your body tissues. The gentle separation of the two surfaces creates a momentary vacuum pop comparable to the sound you make when you stretch a finger and slightly separate your knuckle.

Vertebrae often move, when adjusted, without a

118

sound. The noise does not indicate correction, nor does it help or hinder it; it is just one of the interesting features of the chiropractic adjustment.

Will a back always be weaker after it has been injured?

The body has built-in healing facilities. If you break a bone, the body will try to make that bone as strong as before during the healing process, providing that it is properly set.

Damage your spine and the body will also do its best to restore it to normal, using the correction, mobilization and realignment provided by your chiropractor. Since the spine is a vital body structure, all of the body's healing resources will be marshaled to assist.

Ligamentous tissue heals slowly since it has no direct blood supply. The healing process may take a long time if ligaments are damaged. These are the non-stretching "guy wires" that hold your vertebrae within the normal range of movement. Make sure the ligaments heal completely if you want to achieve full spinal strength again.

Do chiropractors testify in court on their patients' behalf?

Yes. If you are an accident victim, your chiropractor will be able to describe in a legal summary report what he found when he examined you, what he did about it, the extent of your improvement and the degree of ultimate recovery he anticipates. He is qualified as an expert witness to defend his statements in court.

So you're thinking of going to a chiropractor

Is it possible to compare chiropractic and medical treatment of similar injuries?

Studies of the results of treatment have been carried out. In the report of a 1975 conference convened by the National Institute of Neurological Diseases and Stroke, Dr. Ronald Gitelman reported as follows: "An independent research group did an objective review of the Workmen's Compensation Board reports of all cases of spinal strains and sprains in the State of Florida for the year 1956. Cases numbering 19,666 were reviewed by comparing costs and days lost. Under chiropractic care, the average total cost was $60 and days lost were three. Under medical treatment (nonspecialist, nonhospitalization), the average cost was $102 and days lost were nine." (NINDS Monograph No. 15, p. 278).

Is chiropractic becoming more widely used as a means to health?

The 1980 edition of *Who's Who in Chiropractic* contains the following editorial comment: "The emergence of chiropractic into the mainstream of health care is a phenomenon that now evokes more than speculative interest within the academic, social welfare, and scientific communities, as evidenced by a recently federally-funded survey made of the chiropractic profession by the Foundation for the Advancement of Chiropractic Tenets and Science (FACTS). The report, submitted to Congress in March, 1980, projected 'that the number of graduates in the next five years from sixteen chiropractic colleges in the United States will be approximately 13,000 or more than 50 percent of the 26,000 now in practice. . . . The profession's colleges report

120

that they are following a selective admissions policy, with 40 to 60 percent of first-year classes holding baccalaureate degrees. Since 1973 five new chiropractic colleges have been founded.'

"According to FACTS, there were 130 million patient visits to 23,000 practicing DC's (doctors of chiropractic) in the United States during 1979, and in the preceding year the total expenditures on chiropractic care exceeded $1 billion. The report also noted that 41 percent of all such services were provided to individuals in the so-called younger population market—between the ages of 18 and 45.

"Add up these statistics provided by FACTS and one can reasonably envision a bright future for the profession as substantiated by the Dean of the Harvard Medical School who in a projection of medical education into the 1980s predicted '. . . more acceptance for this specialty.' "

Why can a vertebra not be replaced with one powerful correction?

The damage associated with a subluxated vertebra involves more than just the bone. The joints between such vertebrae are affected and movement is often restricted or painful. The muscles and ligaments holding and moving the vertebra are often stretched or out of balance. The nerves which supply the surrounding tissue react and create an abnormal situation. Blood flow is often affected as the brain initiates tissue repair. Swelling is sometimes a factor as tightly packed tissue experiences increased pressure.

A sudden severe correction could in itself create trauma. The gentle chiropractic adjustment persuades

121

the body to return to normal gradually, healing the tissues as they return to their normal functional relationship.

Should an apparently healthy spine ever be manipulated?

Your chiropractor sees every variety of spinal condition in his office. He knows how much trouble spinal distortion and fixation can cause. He knows how internal body organs can be affected by interference with nerve roots at the spine. From time to time he sees a seriously damaged or degenerated spine which is beyond his help.

Ask him how often he has an adjustment to his spine. If his spine feels healthy and pain-free, it is likely that he has an adjustment once every ten to fourteen days. When he is injured or in pain, he will probably be treated every day at least once, possibly twice. He knows how important spinal integrity is to health. He values his health. A healthy spine should be examined regularly to *keep* it healthy.

What is my chiropractor doing when he moves bones in my spine?

Your chiropractor moves spinal bones to restore normal function to spinal nerves and the tissues they serve. This enables the brain to receive accurate information from all body parts. It also enables the body organs and tissues to be completely dominated and controlled by the brain so that body function will be balanced and normal.

He does this in several ways. He corrects the subluxation which he has found in the spinal segment. He checks for the loss of movement between the vertebrae and manipulates to restore any fixation to normal.

122

He also adjusts to correct the juxtaposition of vertebral bodies, if they are crowding too close to each other, so that the space between them will allow normal movement. He is interested in obtaining sufficient free space for the passage of the spinal nerves located behind the vertebral bodies.

What is a subluxation?

A subluxation is defined by the American Chiropractic Association as "the alteration of the normal dynamics, anatomical or physiological relationships of contiguous articular structures." Basically, it is a joint that is not dislocated, but that does have something wrong with it either at rest or in movement.

How is a subluxation found by a chiropractor?

Subluxations are usually found at the time of chiropractic examination. Your chiropractor checks spinal landmarks with his fingers and discovers the malfunction between spinal segments.

Instruments have been developed to confirm the diagnostic findings from palpation. X-ray examination is also used to identify the degree of distortion, the amount of degeneration it has caused and the best corrective approach for the treatment program.

What causes the pain in a subluxated vertebra?

It is not always painful. Some vertebrae are subluxated for a long period of time, only becoming painful when stress is applied to the spine by a reach, a twist or a lift.

The pain often results from irritation of the spinal

123

nerve at the point where it leaves the spine through the intervertebral foramen, the opening between the vertebrae. Irritation to the contents of this foramen may make the nerve react with pain. It may also swell and increase the pressure.

Pain can also result from irritation of the joints where the vertebrae touch each other. Since these joints are not functioning normally, the pressures will be uneven and pain receptors may be activated.

There may also be associated pain in muscles in the area which are put into spasm as a result of the nerve root irritation. Many possibilities for pain exist.

Do chiropractors prescribe drugs in their practice?

Chiropractic treatment is drugless. It is an alternative approach to sickness, disease and injury that stands apart from treatment of patients with drugs. Since many drugs are poisonous substances, your body will surely benefit from avoiding any drugs you do not need. A drug which relieves one problem and in turn causes another must be considered to be of doubtful value.

Some people react strongly to any opposition to the use of drugs. They have become so commonplace in our society that we treat them as friends. Some authorities who have studied drugs extensively have made statements that are worth considering.

Dr. Roger J. Williams is the first biochemist to be elected president of the American Chemical Society. He is a member of the National Academy of Sciences and has received many awards for his research. In his book *Nutrition Against Disease* he writes: "The fact is that medicine has become addicted to the administration of vast quantities of nonbiological medications which I should categorize as dubious or even essentially 'bad.' I am not merely talking about such obvious villains as thalidomide; there are any number of common nonprescription drugs about which I have severe reservations. The basic fault of all these weapons is that they have no known connection with the disease process itself. They tend to mask the difficulty, not eliminate it. They contaminate the internal environment, create dependence on the part of the patient and often complicate the physician's job by erasing valuable clues as to the real source of the trouble."

Dr. Henry G. Bieler practiced medicine for over fifty years, then wrote the book *Food Is Your Best Medicine*. In it he says: "My . . . conclusion is that in almost all cases the use of drugs in treating patients is harmful. Drugs often cause serious side effects and sometimes even create new diseases. The dubious benefits they afford the patient are at the best temporary. Yet the number of drugs on the market increases geometrically every year as each chemical firm develops its own variation of the compounds. The physician is indeed rare who can be completely aware of the potential danger from the side effects of all these drugs."

In 1979 Robert S. Mendelsohn, M.D. wrote *Confessions of a Medical Heretic* while chairman of the Medical Licensing Committee for the State of Illinois and Associate Professor of Preventive Medicine and Community Health in the School of Medicine of the University of Illinois. In his book he says, "Before you take the first dose of any medication your doctor prescribes, you should make it your business to find out more about the drug than your doctor himself knows.

125

Again, learning more about the situation than the doctor won't be all that difficult. Doctors get most of their information about drugs from advertisements and from detail men and their pamphlet handouts. All you have to do is spend some time with a good book or two in order to get the information you need before deciding whether to take a drug or not. The best book to start with is the *Physicians' Desk Reference,* the *PDR.* The *PDR* is the beginning of knowledge about drugs."

He also comments: "You should not let your doctor prescribe a drug without asking him lots of questions. Ask him what will happen if you don't take the drug. Ask him what the drug is supposed to do for you and how it's going to do it. You can ask him the same questions you will bring to the *PDR,* questions about side effects and situations when the drug is not advised. Don't expect too explicit an answer. Most drugs' mechanisms remain mysteries even to the people who develop them. Once you've exposed yourself to all this information, you have to sit down and decide whether or not you want to take the drug."

Eric W. Martin, in his monumental work *Hazards of Medication,* gives the following information: "There are no harmless medications. All are potentially hazardous to some extent and all must be prescribed and administered with caution. Otherwise patients may be seriously injured. . . . In the United States alone, some 1,500,000 of the 30,000,000 patients hospitalized annually are admitted because of adverse reactions to drugs.

"In some hospitals, as high as 20 percent of the patients are admitted because of drug-induced disease and during the one-year period beginning July 1, 1965 at the Montreal General Hospital, 25 percent of the deaths on the public medical service were the result of adverse drug reaction.

"In five Boston, Massachusetts, institutions, during one two-year period about 31 percent (778) of a group (2514) of hospitalized medical patients experienced adverse drug reactions, of which 80 percent were major or moderately severe.

"During one three-month period of surveillance at Johns Hopkins Hospital, 17 percent (122 of 714) of the general medical service patients experienced 184 adverse drug reactions. This was an incidence of 150 percent and most of the patients (80 percent or 97 of 122) acquired their reactions during the period of hospitalization. Over 30 percent of the patients who were hospitalized evidencing a drug reaction (36 of 122) acquired another reaction in the hospital and of this group 22 percent (8 of 36) died either from the reaction that caused their admission or from one acquired in the hospital after admission."

Do chiropractors take the Hippocratic Oath like medical doctors?

No. Chiropractors take the Chiropractic Oath which takes into consideration Hippocrates' noteworthy observation which has been recorded for posterity: "Look well to the spine for the cause of disease."

The text of the Chiropractic Oath is as follows:

"I do hereby swear before God and these assembled witnesses, both corporeal and spiritual, that I will do my utmost to keep this, my sacred, trusted oath, as a graduate of ――― College, that henceforth:

"I will esteem those who taught me this Art, Science, and Philosophy of Chiropractic and with this torch fashioned by Hippocrates, I will light the way to the understanding of those Natural Laws which preserve the human body as a fitting temple for the soul of man.

"I will keep the physical, mental and spiritual needs of the sick as my foremost duty, ever searching for and correcting the cause of their disease to the best of my ability, insofar as my science is in the highest precepts of my Alma Mater and harmonious with the *Vis Medicatrix Naturae*.

"I will at all times stand ready to serve my fellow man, without distinction of race, creed or color, in my lifelong vocation of preventing and alleviating human suffering wherever it may be found, by exemplifying in my own life a pattern of living in harmony with the laws of nature.

"I will refrain from any act of wrongdoing and will regard the keeping of a patient's confidence as a moral obligation, using any such information in his or her best interests.

"May God so direct the skillful use of my hands that I may bring strength to the sick, relief to the suffering, peace of mind to the anxious and the inspiration of mankind to attain bountiful health that we may live this life to the fullest expression of its innate endowments. I therefore solemnly swear to uphold those principles and precepts to the best of my ability, so help me God."

Where does chiropractic fit in the scientific community?

Chiropractic is the second largest primary health care profession in North America. It is based on principles that are now widely understood. No scientific body would disagree with the concept that the nervous system controls body cells and systems, or that impaired function of the nervous system seriously affects the health of the body. Chiropractors manipulate the spinal bones to free nerves from irritation so they can get their work done without interference.

A Royal Commission in New Zealand studied chiropractic in 1979 and published its findings in a book, *Chiropractic in New Zealand*. In the "Summary of Principal Findings" the Commission states, "Chiropractors should, in the public interest, be accepted as partners in the general health care system. No other health professional is as well qualified by his general training to carry out a diagnosis for spinal mechanical dysfunction or to perform spinal manual therapy."

Does the chiropractic adjustment hurt?

The chiropractic adjustment to the spine is given in such a way that as few pain sensors as possible are activated. When a spine that has no pain is adjusted, the manipulation is pleasant. Afterwards the patient has a relaxed sensation. Some describe it as the way you feel after a stretch or a deep yawn.

When the spine is in trouble and a nerve root is swollen and tender, the chiropractor opens the space, gently, easing the pressure away from the nerve. This causes some minor discomfort. After the first visit, most patients return for chiropractic correction without apprehension.

Can my chiropractor guarantee results?

Chiropractic has grown to its present prominence on the basis of results alone. No chiropractor wants a single failure.

129

So you're thinking of going to a chiropractor

Before you commence chiropractic treatment, your chiropractor should tell you what he expects to be able to do for you. He bases this on his study and experience as applied to the findings in your case. He is not selling cures. Rather, he will chart the road back to good health for you and will do his utmost to remove the roadblocks in your way.

Beware of the person who promises to cure you. I once heard a respected chiropractor explain to a patient, "If anyone ever promises you a cure, that's the time to start running."

Will my chiropractor give me a massage?

No. When the spine is adjusted, much of the muscle tension is relieved. The muscles respond to the normal control of the nerves that serve them. If your chiropractor finds a muscle that is in spasm, or that is too relaxed, he will use a muscle technique to correct the situation.

Do chiropractors refer patients to medical doctors?

Yes. When an examination shows that a problem exists which chiropractic cannot help, it is your chiropractor's responsibility to refer you to the person you need to see. There are specific legal boundaries to each health discipline which must be rigidly observed.

A patient came to my office a few days ago with extreme back pain. Examination suggested the existence of serious injury, and X-ray examination showed spinal fracture. She was advised of our findings and sent for the medical supervision she required.

Questions patients ask their chiropractors

Do chiropractors ever advise surgery?

Surgery is sometimes necessary in severe back cases. Your chiropractor will discuss this with you. If you require surgery, he will refer you to a surgeon in whom he has confidence, based on experience.

Dr. Andrew B. Wymore, a Kansas chiropractor, chaired the Therapeutic Studies section of the National Institute of Neurological Diseases and Stroke conference on Spinal Manipulative Therapy in 1975 in Bethesda, Maryland. In his Chairman's Summary he stated: "At one time statistics indicated that fusion was a good form of treatment for low back pain, and this is no longer the case. . . . Studies from Mayo Clinic, Philadelphia (from Rothman) and Seattle, Washington have demonstrated that lumbar fusion is not the operation for low back pain and that it is being abandoned in the United States. In Sweden it was given up some ten years ago."

A person is wise to consider all the alternatives before deciding to undergo spinal surgery. It is also wise to have more than one surgical assessment. The result of surgery is not always dramatic relief. Ask your chiropractor how often he is asked for help by a person in pain, although the patient has already experienced a spinal surgical procedure.

Why do health professionals not work as a team?

To a great extent they do. The patient is always uppermost in the thinking of the health care practitioner, whatever his field. I have had many referrals from professionals who would have preferred to continue with the cases, but the patient came first in their thinking.

131

So you're thinking of going to a chiropractor

The human body is extremely complex. Training in the healing professions is specific, intricate and detailed. The practitioner, having mastered his own discipline, tends to feel that he is the only one who knows how. The struggle for excellence is good for the patient, but it sometimes fosters criticism of others and their methods.

This interprofessional crossfire is sometimes misunderstood by the patient. There is nothing personal about it. Professional people know their own field but they are not always tuned in to what another professional is doing. Persons with a different method become suspect, even though they are extremely proficient.

Do chiropractors ever treat babies?

Yes. Chiropractors often treat babies in the first week of life, and on through the childhood years. Special techniques are used during infancy to overcome the trauma of childbirth.

Why does a chiropractor still feel the spine after he has taken X-rays?

The X-rays give an accurate picture of your spine as of the time they were made, but you are a moving and changing person. As correction is given, there is a change of muscle balance as the body adapts to the correction and returns to more normal vertebral relationships. Your chiropractor's fingers assure him that the adjustments to the spine are effective. They also tell him if any underlying problem is presenting itself. He is in touch with the changes.

A leading educator in chiropractic, Dr. H. O. Beatty, wrote in his book *Anatomical Adjustive Technic:* "The work of the chiropractor is centered to a great

132

extent in his hands. Through palpation of the patient, we consider diagnostic signs of relationship, size, shape, density, resistance, tonicity, texture, temperature, movement and indirectly, sensation."

When should I use ice on a back injury?

Use ice when your chiropractor advises it. He is in touch with your individual problem, and can tailor his advice to your situation. The general rule is to use ice when the problem is acute and swelling in any of the tissues is a possibility.

What are the side effects of chiropractic adjustments?

There are virtually no side effects to chiropractic adjustments unless increased flexibility, diminishing pain, or relaxation of muscle tension can be considered side effects. Sometimes, during a series of corrective adjustments, stiffness or pain in a new area will be noticed by the patient, but this transitory experience is the body's reaction to necessary inner changes required for the restoration of body balance. Nothing is added to the body and nothing is taken from it. When your condition has been diagnosed by your chiropractor as calling for controlled chiropractic correction, this treatment has no hazards for the patient. This is a unique feature of chiropractic. Medical textbooks now describe a substantial number of what are called iatrogenic diseases—diseases caused by medicines administered for other conditions. Chiropractic has no such listings—and, for that matter, chiropractic malpractice insurance fees are low indeed, a fact which speaks for itself.

So you're thinking of going to a chiropractor

Can a person with arthritis take chiropractic adjustments?

Yes. Chiropractors adjust arthritic patients every day in practice. Every body tissue benefits from normal nerve function and control. There is also the added benefit of moving the joints of the spine and extremities through their normal range of motion. Your chiropractor will also advise you on the proper nutritional approach to your condition and the use of heat and cold at home.

Do chiropractors treat disc problems?

Yes. When a disc is first injured, a swelling takes place which may press against a spinal nerve and cause extreme pain with muscle spasms in the area of injury as the body works to splint the weakened area. Your chiropractor will use every means at his disposal to reduce the swelling, open up the disc space, correct the associated distortion and restore the normal movement to the injured area of the spine. If you talk with some of his patients, you will find that his track record is good. Disc injuries require longer supervision than many other spinal problems. After the pain is gone, great care needs to be taken to prevent reinjury or degenerative changes in the disc.

What is meant by a slipped disc?

This is loose terminology. Discs do not slip. Sometimes the edge of the disc cracks open in an injury, allowing the soft center of the disc to pass out. The disc is then said to be herniated or ruptured. More often the disc swells and bulges, and the bulging disc substance presses against a spinal nerve, causing great pain.

134

What should I do to speed my recovery from a low back injury?

Here are a few general rules which will assist your chiropractor to get you pain-free as quickly as possible while he corrects your problem and then brings a measure of stability to your spine.

Do no lifting until your chiropractor approves it.

Use the balance of rest and activity your chiropractor advises.

Ask your chiropractor how you should sleep to help yourself.

Avoid constipation. Bearing down is hurtful.

Let walking be your major exercise.

For prolonged standing, put one foot on a step or book ahead of you.

If you sit to watch TV, walk around during the commercials.

Avoid soft chairs and soft beds.

Avoid uneven ground.

Wear slip-free footwear in snow or ice.

Apply no heat until your chiropractor specifically advises it.

When you bend forward at the waist, bend your knees slightly.

Support your back when you cough or sneeze—lean against your hand.

On trips, stop and walk around the car every half hour.

What causes subluxations in the spine?

They may be caused by a fall or bump, by a twist, a lift, a stretch or a sudden move in sleep. We cause subluxations by sitting incorrectly at a desk, by bending in an awkward position, by losing our balance and getting it again, and by reacting suddenly to a shock or fright. They result from swinging a golf club carelessly, from stress or worry, from stepping accidentally off a curb or step and jerking ourselves, or from sneezing. A cold draft on a muscle may also cause a subluxation. There are many causes.

Why should I worry about subluxations if my back is not hurting?

A subluxation is always a problem to the body, even though it may not raise the pain signal to get our attention. A subluxation creates a situation which will result in abnormal functioning. It is a stepping-stone to future pain and potential illness. Your spine should receive the same attention you would give any other part of your body that was known to be in trouble.

Since a subluxation in the spine is out of sight, we may put it out of mind for a while. Chiropractors see evidence every day that convinces them that a subluxation should not be ignored, even when there is no pain. Spinal nerves that pass from the spine through a subluxation will sooner or later give notice that they are irritated by the distortion.

17

Chiropractic for athletes— and everyone

ATHLETES are part of every chiropractor's practice. At every level of participation the tennis player, golfer, football hero, gymnast or skier puts the added strain on the body which is the price of being a winner. Any misalignment in a body pushed to perform at such a peak is bound to create stress and ultimately become a problem.

The chiropractor often sees the athlete after the injury, but his best contribution is made when he has the opportunity to align and balance body structures before the game or competition.

Groups of chiropractors in different parts of the world have developed programs of care for the contenders in every athletic pursuit, and the volume of results is expanding steadily.

Dr. Leroy Perry, Jr. is a leader in this thrust. With his team of associates, he cares for a large cross-section of world-class athletes, using specialized techniques developed during the last decade. Dr. Perry formed the Foundation for Athletic Research and Education, based in West Los Angeles, in association with basketball great Wilt Chamberlain, Vernon Wolfe, head track coach at the University of Southern California, and a number of other professionals concerned with the care and wellbeing of athletes. Their goal is to do investigative research into the prevention and alleviation of athletic and stress-related injuries. F.A.R.E. is dedicated to the advancement of athletic potential in men and women of all ages.

The staff of consultants working with F.A.R.E. includes coaches, Olympic and professional athletes, chiropractors, dentists, podiatrists, physicians, athletic trainers, nutritionists, kinesiologists, psychologists, exercise physiologists, biochemical and computer stress analysts, sports anthropologists, biofeedback experts and other highly trained technicians.

The techniques developed by Dr. Perry and his associates were so effective in caring for athletes that the news spread and soon leaders in sports were flying across the country for treatment. It soon became evident that the time had come to teach the perfected

138

methods to chiropractors across the continent and to have regular updating programs to keep them in touch with the continuing new developments of the program.

The Institute for Sports Therapy and Rehabilitation was established. In 1982 and 1983 thirty-two teaching seminars were planned and conducted in eight major cities across the United States from New York to Los Angeles. The invitation to attend was accompanied by notes from twenty-six of Dr. Perry's patients who had been treated with the methods developed by himself and his team. The names read like a *Who's Who* of the athletic and entertainment worlds, including Amy Alcott, Tracy Austin, Willie Banks, Warren Beatty, Ricky Bell, Ron Cey, Wilt Chamberlain, James Coburn, Susan Clark, Patty Reagan Davis, Doug DeCinces, Mariel Hemingway, Alex Karras, Shelly Mann, Ricardo Montalban, John Naber, Jack Nicholson, Murray Rose, James Sanford, Doc Severinsen, William Shatner, Stan Smith, Dwight Stones, Toni Tennille, Mac Wilkin and Donna Caponna Young.

When I attended the I-STAR seminar in New York City, I mentioned to Dr. Perry my interest in sharing some of the principles he applies to athletes in this book. His positive response was immediate. He pointed out that the factors which enable athletes to reduce stress and perform at peak efficiency will help the average person enjoy more abundant health, with less wear from stress.

It is possible for the body to become more efficient if there is balance in its movements. When this balance of activity is present, we are less prone to be injured, even when a sudden unusual strain is placed upon us, as in a fall or twist.

139

So you're thinking of going to a chiropractor

There are three vital factors in this balance. The mind plans where we want to go, outlines the steps to take to get there and handles the disappointments and defeats on the way. The body is the unit of action and must be structurally sound, with the parts mechanically aligned and a movement pattern that maintains the alignment rather than disrupts it. The biochemical link between mind and body is nutrition, which must supply essential factors for the maintenance of each body part while at the same time providing energy at the rate required for peak performance.

There are certain principles of body movement that can bring out the hidden athlete in each of us. Posture is the basis of it, but it must be posture that is present whether we sit, walk, stand or run.

Since our feet are the foundation of our activity, their placement is important. The body works most efficiently if we learn to place our feet so that they are almost parallel, with the center of the heel directly behind the joint between the first and second toes. This is the normal placing of our feet in any activity, and allows efficient ankle, knee and hip activity. By making this one simple change in your stance you will have started toward more healthy movement.

Correct foot placement takes practice and concentration over a period of time. You must overcome established habits. Keep in mind that a youthful appearance has good posture as part of it. Posture tends to deteriorate with age, unless we decide to do something about it. Watch people walking toward you on a busy sidewalk and you will see this for yourself.

The next basic area is the pelvis. Through the years we have been told to pull the abdomen in, but it is

140

much more effective, and better for the whole body stance, to pull the pubis up toward the navel. This is a natural, easy action which can be developed quickly into habit because it is pleasant rather than uncomfortable, and takes pressure off the low back.

Once the foot placement and pubis elevation are mastered, a third location for concentration is the breastbone, midway between the nipples. This point on the sternum should be held at the highest comfortable level. Breathing capacity will increase, the slightly stretched abdomen will flatten and the rib cage and the thoracic spine will function more efficiently.

Then concentrate on the top of your head. Hold it high for the most efficient functioning of all neck and upper back structures. Many people tuck the neck into the shoulders when rising from a sitting position. The best function is attained when the neck is extended to its greatest length.

Dr. Perry stimulates the imagination by suggesting that we should imagine helium-filled balloons attached to the pubis, the mid-sternum and the top of our heads, pulling at full strength. Sounds simple, but it works. Athletes, actors and actresses, musicians, businessmen and many chiropractors whom I know personally have benefited from this simple application of imagery.

Bill Malincheck of the Washington Redskins told me that after the third game every year he used to expect to play for the rest of the season with pain. Though he had suffered some serious injuries, chiropractic correction and a practical application of some of the basics outlined here have given him productive rather than pain-filled years.

141

So you're thinking of going to a chiropractor

Now that you understand the positioning of the body while standing with efficient posture, it is important to consider balance. Many of us stand with our weight on our heels, our knees locked back and our abdomen forward. The correct body stance will put the center of weight distribution slightly ahead of the ankle. This is accomplished by tilting the body ever so slightly forward while envisioning the three balloons at work. You will notice that the metatarsal arch of the foot starts to feel its portion of the weight, the leg muscles are more active, which helps the return of blood in the veins of the legs, and the heel does not register much weight. It is an action stance that will not quickly fatigue you.

Dr. Perry has a colorful posture suggestion in *F.A.R.E. Play* magazine: "What is your favorite color? Blue? Every time you see the color blue, or any derivative of blue, imagine the balloons filling with more helium. As a result, your pelvis starts to lift, your neck elongates, you feel taller. As your pelvis lifts, your back will become less tense; as your chest rises, your shoulders and upper back relax; and as your head lifts, the back of your neck relaxes. . . . So pick your favorite color balloon and begin. Remember what Albert Einstein said: 'Imagination is more important than knowledge.' "

Proper walking is accomplished by tilting the balanced body forward about five degrees and pushing off with the back foot. The forward foot will touch ground about three-quarters of an inch in front of the heel. The arms will swing forward and backward with no side deviation. Eyes will look ahead, not on the ground. The three helium balloons are still pulling the pubis, the sternum and the top of the head. You will love walking when you learn this technique. It is bio-efficient, and you will be aware of the ease with which you cover the ground. Remember to push with the rear foot, not pull with the forward foot, and keep the body balance slightly forward as you walk.

Running requires a forward angle of ten to twenty degrees. It is still a pushing action, with the foot touching the ground about three-quarters of an inch ahead of the heel. Arms must move in pendulum fashion with no side swing, no higher than nipple level in front and slightly above hip level behind. Feel the pull of the three balloons as you run. Keep hands and jaw relaxed. Your stride will be lengthened by proper positioning of the pelvis.

As you put these principles into practice, you will notice the change in your movements and your appearance. The simplicity of it may make you grow careless and slip into the old way of standing and walking. It will take long-term practice and concentration to make good posture a way of life.

I watched video programs of Tracy Austin being taught to walk and run by Dr. Perry. She was already a tennis pro with a string of winning accomplishments behind her. It was no secret that her injuries were threatening her future in tennis. Dr. Perry taught her how to walk with such alignment that her movements were bio-efficient. She worked at it like the winner she is. Running was added to her program of corrective supervision only after she had mastered walking. As she ran back and forward across the tennis court, the change in her control was evident. Further training in the balancing and coordination of the muscles of the back, shoulder and chest was given by Dr. Perry.

143

Structurally and functionally in alignment, Tracy went to Japan to win again. In her own words: "Dr. Leroy Perry's help enabled me to win—when others could not."

18

The tomorrow of chiropractic

THE wide public attention paid to research into cancer, heart disease and the other great killers makes many of us forget that research is a part of every health discipline, including chiropractic. Chiropractic rarely deals with dramatically immediate life-threatening conditions, but what has developed from its practice and its research programs directly affects the quality of the life we live, not just its length.

I inquired of Dr. Howard Vernon, Director of the Research Board of the Canadian Memorial Chiropractic College, and found that the college had local research programs in progress at the college facility; and in various parts of Canada satellite activities are under way.

In the last seven years, C.M.C.C. has sponsored three major studies into the effect of chiropractic treatment on low back pain. The first study was initiated in Saskatoon in 1977 at the University Hospital in association with Dr. Kirkaldy Willis, an orthopedic surgeon of considerable repute in his field. This was a five-year study of in-patients with low back pain. Their response to manipulation was investigated. A second similar study was initiated in 1981 by C.M.C.C. at McMaster's Chedoke Hospital in association with their chief of neurology, Dr. Adrian Upton. The third study was conducted on the C.M.C.C. campus. A Low Back Pain Clinic was established in 1982 to engage in advanced care and research of low back pain sufferers.

A second focus of clinical research has been headaches. There is a major study already under way to determine the effect of chiropractic on migraine in adults.

In the area of biomechanics, C.M.C.C. has developed a unique Posture/Gait Laboratory for the study of the human spine and locomotor system. Research into diagnostic and therapeutic applications of gait and posture study is being carried on in this facility. Many techniques of spinal analysis which are unique to chiropractors are being investigated constantly.

Several studies of the physiological effects of manipulation are in progress. The object is to determine whether manipulation affects the body's levels of cortisone, endorphins, melatonin and glucose. Several of these studies are being conducted in association with Toronto's Banting Institute Laboratory.

Neurophysiological studies have been done demonstrating that manipulation affects nerve conduction and reflex activity of the spinal cord and increases pain thresholds around the spine.

Basic science research is being conducted by chiropractors into:

1) the effect of electrical stimulation of bone growth, at Toronto's Sunnybrook Hospital;

2) the autoimmune reaction in the intervertebral disc, at the University of Toronto;

3) a small-animal model of spinal subluxation, at Sunnybrook Hospital; and

4) a small-animal model study of the biochemistry of the arthritic reaction, at the University of Toronto.

C.M.C.C. also researches products for employers and suppliers. The present studies are quite varied. Under a Canada Post grant, a new strap is being designed for letter carriers. A new device to produce inverted traction in the sitting position for relief of backache is being studied. Water beds and their effects on the spine and spinal pain are under examination.

A computer database is being established for the chiropractic profession. The goal of the team is to have every bit of chiropractic literature in the world indexed and available to anyone involved in chiropractic research.

And all this research is associated with a single college. Think of the number of chiropractic colleges in the United States and around the world, each with its own program of scientific investigative research! More cooperation from centers of scientific research is being offered, as results need to be duplicated by various groups to confirm and advance the findings.

Dr. Robert A. Leach wrote a synopsis of scientific research into chiropractic which he titled *The Chiropractic Theories*. He states:

> Late in the last decade, C. H. Suh came to the conclusion, following some personal investigation, that the chiropractic profession needed not only broad clinical studies but basic research. The University of Colorado professor soon came under pressure from colleagues, government officials, and health professionals to abandon the idea of initiating basic chiropractic research even before he had begun. Yet Suh went on to organize a program of study which has evolved into the area of biomechanics, neurophysiology, and neurochemistry. These studies have been funded by the university itself, the International Chiropractors' Association (ICA), the American Chiropractic Association (ACA), and the Federal Government.
>
> In addition, interdisciplinary conferences have resulted in a virtual renaissance of research for the chiropractic profession in this decade. Scott Haldeman has formed the International Society for the Advancement of Clinical Chiropractic and Spinal Research. An ACA-sponsored organization, the Foundation for Chiropractic Education and Research, operates out of Des Moines, Iowa. An ICA-sponsored organization, the Foundation for the Advancement of Chiropractic Tenets and Science, is based in Washington, D.C.
>
> The various chiropractic colleges have been instrumental in promoting studies through the years. B. J. Palmer, at the Palmer School of Chiropractic, supervised many experiments on subluxation and was even

148

responsible for some of the comparison studies involving chiropractic versus medical care. Joseph Janse, at the National College of Chiropractic, has promoted chiropractic for decades and helped Dr. Illi with some of his basic research into spinal mechanics.

The work of Dr. Illi in Geneva, Switzerland centered on the mechanics of spinal movement. As Director of the Institute for the Study of the Mechanics, Statics, and Dynamics of the Human Body, he had special equipment made so that he could X-ray the body in every possible position, stressed and unstressed.

Illi was able to show that when the sacroiliac was subluxated on one side only, the fifth lumbar was consistently involved. He also did work with the center of mobile gravity, plotting it by use of a four-point scale that could read the weight resting on the front and rear of each foot. He developed specialized equipment for research into the treatment of scoliosis and to exercise the sacroiliac joints equally or with the emphasis on one of the joints.

Dr. Illi's work was so exacting that in his intense research into pelvic movement he would take a dissected human specimen in the lab and make as many as 100 X-rays of the movement of joints, moving only two or three degrees at a time; then he would take photographs of the resulting X-rays. The still photographs were then used to make a movie of the action of the pelvis so that detailed study of the movement could be made.

One of the problems in research involving spinal adjustment is the need for a pretended adjustment. This requires to have a control group of people who think they were adjusted but were not. It is easy to give a

placebo such as sugar pill to a control group in a drug
research project, but how can an adjustment be given
and yet not given? This obstacle has yet to be overcome.

The dilemma reminds me of the fact that my
office is just a few city blocks from the famed Shute
Institute where so much work was done with vitamin
E. Much of Dr. Shute's work was rejected because he
refused to have a control group who thought they were
getting vitamin E for their hearts when they were not.
He said he would not let people die to prove a point.

In 1976 Dr. Joseph Janse wrote a foreword to an
collection of his writings compiled by Dr. R.W. Hilde-
brand, *Principles and Practice of Chiropractic,* in which he
says:

> Future research efforts in chiropractic should con-
> sider the following:
>
> 1. The search for new knowledge of man as a whole
> organism in which all structures and functions are
> reciprocally integrated for the benefit of the body as a
> whole.
>
> 2. The search for the specific relationship between bio-
> chemical disorders of the musculoskeletal system and
> the functional integrity of other systems of the body.
>
> 3. The search for the intimate relationship of spinal
> and pelvic articular derangements to disturbances of the
> related neurological elements.
>
> 4. The study of physiologic unity of the body, and of
> health and disease as a natural condition.
>
> 5. The study of the adaptation of skeletal muscle to sus-
> tained tension—active and passive—and the effects
> mirrored reflexly in the autonomic and somatic ner-
> vous system components.

6. The study of nutrition as it relates to nerve tissue and the effects of nutritional deficiencies on neurological function.

7. The study of the incidence and effects of spinal and pelvic developmental defects.

All of these, and other studies, by their very nature will not lead to cures for specific diseases, nor are they pursued with specific diseases in mind. Certainly, however, a thorough investigation of them will lead to an increased knowledge in areas of human affliction about which so little is actually now known.

Many procedures in the healing arts are changing, as a method or technique is replaced by one that is better. Almost ninety years have passed since the first chiropractic adjustment was given.

New methods have been developed through research and experience with millions of patients, but the years have shown the consistent benefit to sick and injured people from spinal manipulation by the world's chiropractors. The basic concept of restoring normal function to tissue through manipulation of the spine has not changed, however that manipulation is accomplished.

Chiropractic continues to expand as more thinking people are looking for an approach to health that uses natural laws and principles that are not in themselves harmful or dangerous. The chiropractor sees daily in his office those people who have been told that nothing further can be done or that they must learn to live with the pain. He enjoys turning it around for these people. This is the challenge of his profession. He knows that everything has not been done if chiropractic has not been included.

151

Appendix

Medical acceptance of chiropractic

MEDICAL opposition to chiropractic has all too often been the rule, but more and more medical doctors have by observation and experience come to adopt a different position. Here are some recent comments of this sort.

Two medical doctors, W. B. Parsons and J. D. A. Cummings, wrote in the *Canadian Medical Association Journal* as long ago as July 1958, "The reason we took up manipulation was an interest in backache, with the early discovery that many patients who failed to respond to routine medical treatment went to a manipulator and received immediate relief. This discovery was followed by acceptance of the classic advice, 'If you can't whip 'em, join 'em,' at least to the extent of borrowing their techniques."

Later, in September, 1964, Hoyle Campbell, M.D., Associate Professor of Surgery at the University of Toronto, gave an address to the College of General Practitioners of Canada and was reported by the *Globe and Mail* to have said: "Pain referred from neck muscles to the chest may even be diagnosed as angina [by the physician], so that the patient goes in fear of his life and becomes ill from the stress of his fears. Such a man may then go to a manipulator and be cured."

The *Ontario Medical Review* carried comments in its February, 1966 issue by W. D. Thomas, M.D., as follows: "The young family doctor soon learns that backache and malfunctioning joints, about which he heard so little during his training, are very common complaints. Very little is taught in the medical schools about mechanical lesions of the spine or locomotor systems, and nothing whatever about manipulation. The average doctor in general practice confesses to complete lack of knowledge on the subject. . . . For many years it has been most embarrassing to find that our patients would drift off to lay manipulators, where sometimes they experienced rather spectacular cures, much to the embarrassment of organized medicine."

Ronald Barber, a medical doctor from England, addressed the Toronto Academy of Medicine and commented, "Seventeen percent of my patients require manipulation, and it is a tragic fact that the average physician learns of manipulation after his patient has been helped by someone outside the medical profession. This naturally arouses resentment."

S. S. B. Gilder, another medical doctor, made a statement in the May, 1964 issue of the *Canadian Medical Association Journal:* "Teachers of medical students know little of indications for or contraindications to manipulation, or its technique, and therefore cannot teach it. Thus the young practitioner may be irritated to find that his un-manipulated patients have sought relief from a layman and may project his irritation onto manipulation rather than his ignorance."

In New Zealand, a Royal Commission took a long hard look at chiropractic in 1979 and published a 377-page report which is available for general purchase from the Government Printer, Wellington, New Zealand. Following are a few of the statements in their "Summary of Principal Findings."

> Modern chiropractic is far from being an "un-scientific cult."
>
> Chiropractic is a branch of the healing arts specializing in the correction by spinal manipulation therapy of what chiropractors identify as biomechanical disorders of the spinal column. They carry out spinal diagnosis and therapy at a sophisticated and refined level.
>
> Chiropractors are the only health practitioners who are necessarily equipped by their education and training to carry out spinal manual therapy.
>
> General medical practitioners and physiotherapists have no adequate training in spinal manual

155

therapy, though a few have acquired skill in it subsequent to graduation.

Spinal manual therapy in the hands of a registered chiropractor is safe.

The education and training of a registered chiropractor are sufficient to enable him to determine whether there are contraindications to spinal manual therapy in a particular case, and whether the patient should have medical care instead of or as well as chiropractic care.

Spinal manual therapy can be effective in relieving musculoskeletal symptoms such as back pain, and other symptoms known to respond to such therapy, such as migraine.

In a limited number of cases where there are organic and/or visceral symptoms, chiropractic treatment may provide relief, but this is unpredictable, and in such cases the patient should be under concurrent medical care if that is practicable.

Although the precise nature of the biomechanical dysfunction which chiropractors claim to treat has not yet been demonstrated scientifically, and although the precise reasons why spinal manual therapy provides relief have not yet been scientifically explained, chiropractors have reasonable grounds based on clinical evidence for their belief that symptoms of the kind described above can respond beneficially to spinal manual therapy.

Three sociologists, specializing in the study of health and health care, each of them university professors with experience in health field research, studied chiropractic in depth. The 300-page report of findings of the study by Professors M. Kelner, O. Hall and I. Coulter was published by Fitzhenry and Whiteside

Ltd. in 1980. Their postscript contains the following comments:

> Chiropractic offers to the patient holistic care; it goes beyond treatment to the total management of a patient's case, as well as offering advice on the prevention of future problems and maintenance of good health. It offers the patient conservative care; chiropractors use low-risk procedures aimed at conserving health, and avoid treatment that may have negative side effects. It offers available care; chiropractic is characterized by available offices, spread throughout large urban centers and small rural communities. Chiropractors also make a point of being available to their patients, starting early in the morning and working late in the evening, and assuring patients of their continuing availability when terminating their case. Chiropractic offers immediate care; no prolonged testing is required before treatment can begin. Moreover, chiropractic care usually yields early relief and often provides early restoration of functioning. It offers personal care; chiropractors approach their patients with a personal orientation and personalized attitudes. Their concern is for the whole person, not the limb or the "case." It offers intelligible care; chiropractors try to provide their patients with an understanding of their injury or illness, using language which patients can comprehend. They explain the plan of treatment, the progress of the case, and the relation of their illness to environmental conditions. Finally, they try to make their patients aware of their personal role and responsibility in the maintenance of their own health. Chiropractic is cooperative care—patients participate as partners in the treatment and enhancing of their own health.
>
> In summary then, chiropractic's claim to distinc-

157

tion rests on the fact that it is holistic, conservative, available, immediate, personal, intelligible, and cooperative. These features largely explain why, in the course of this study, patients expressed such a high level of satisfaction.